Connectivity and Functional Specialization in the Brain

Edited by Thomas Heinbockel and Yongxia Zhou

Published in London, United Kingdom

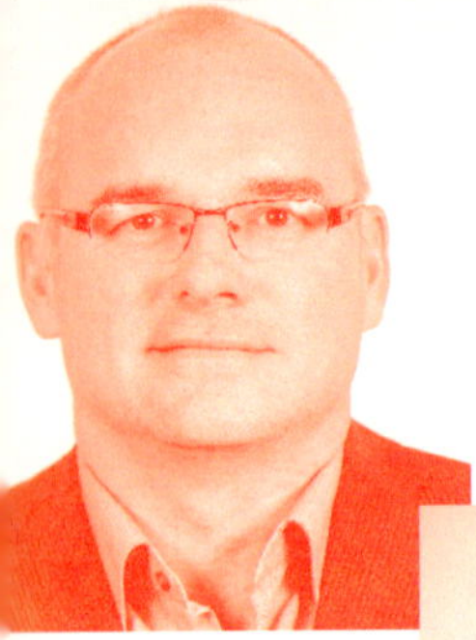
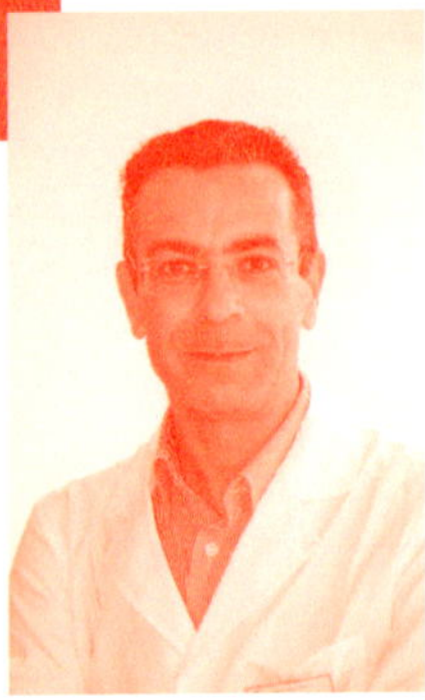
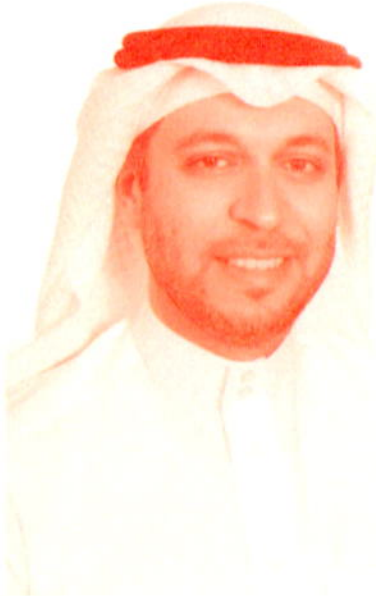
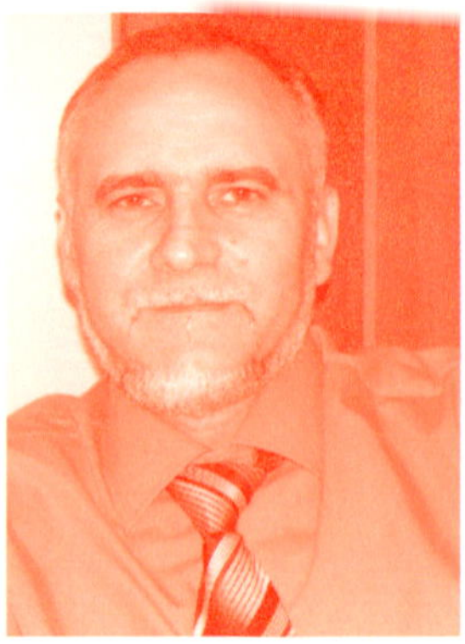
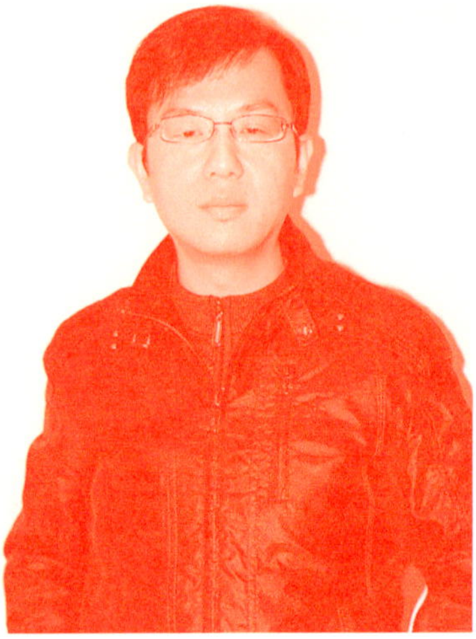
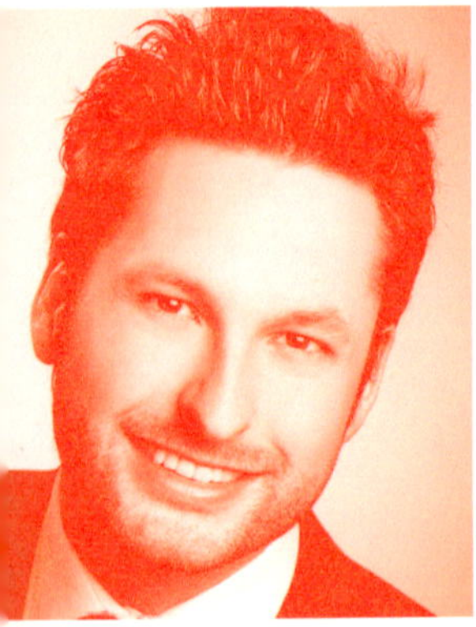
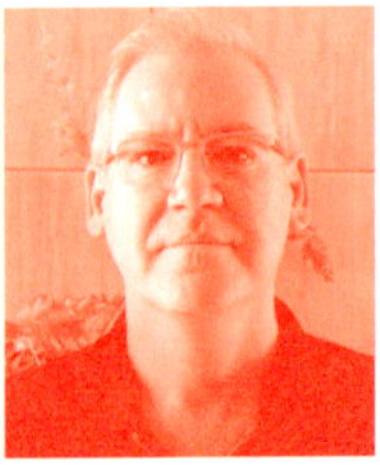

IntechOpen

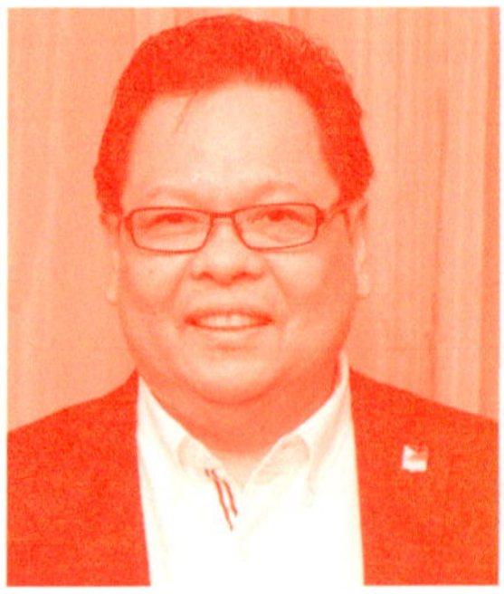
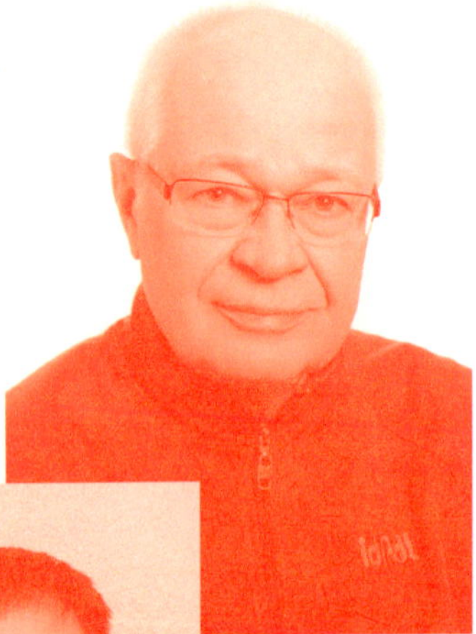
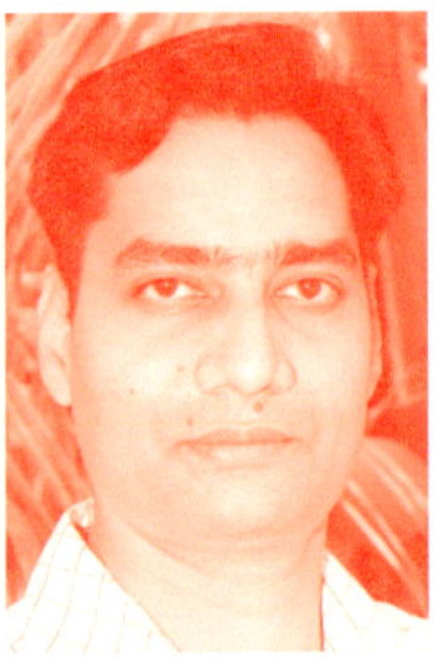
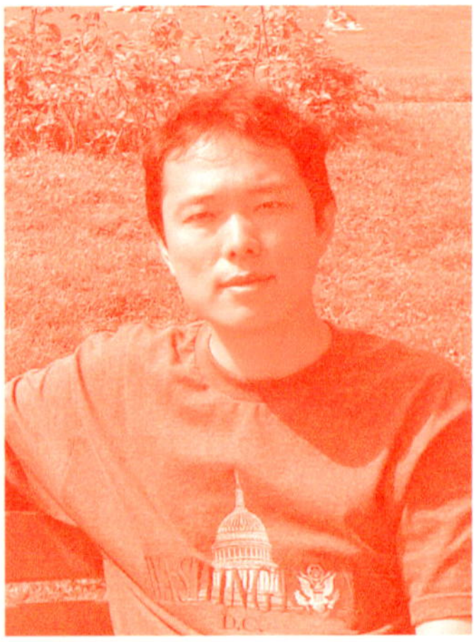
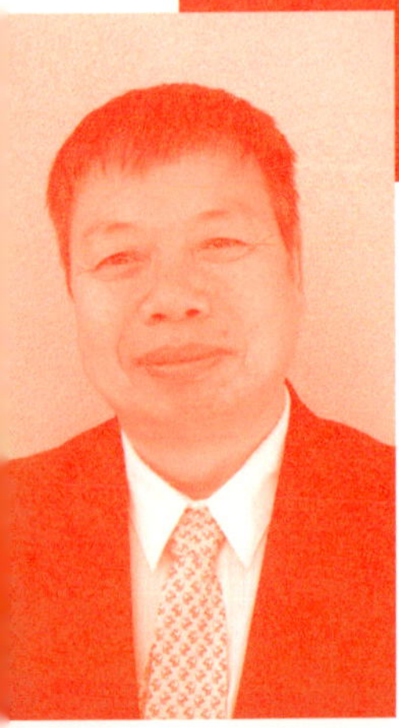
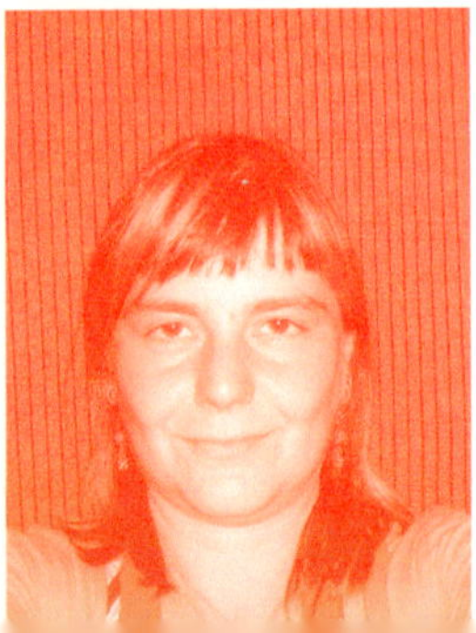

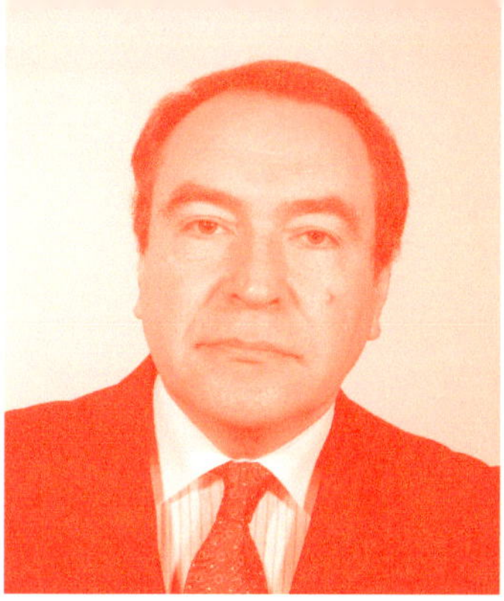

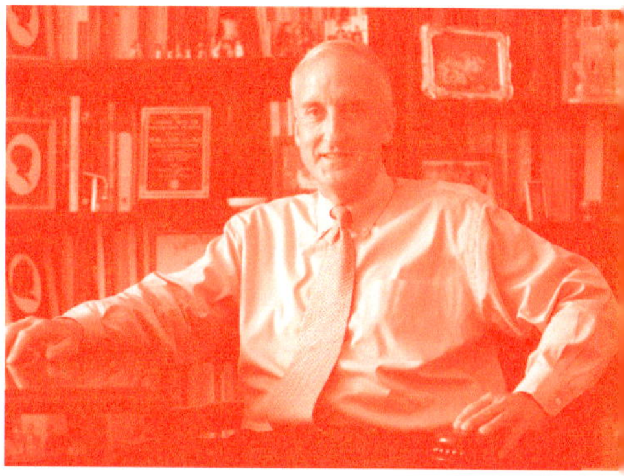

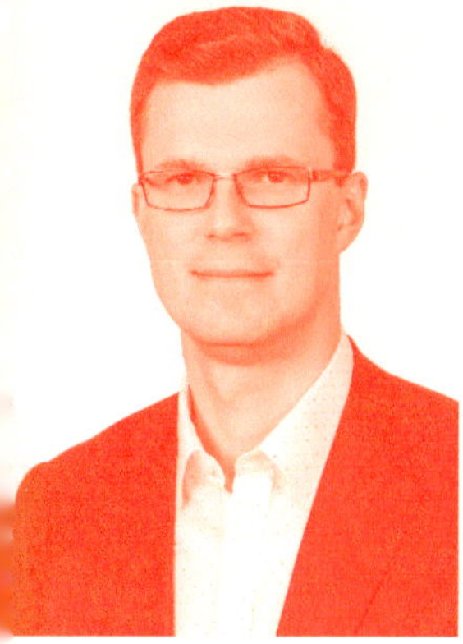

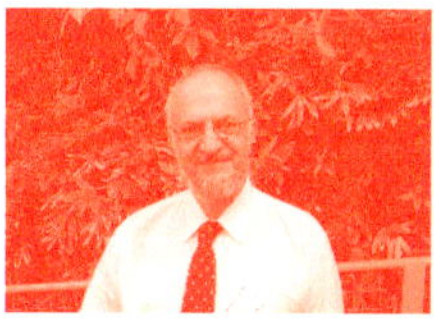

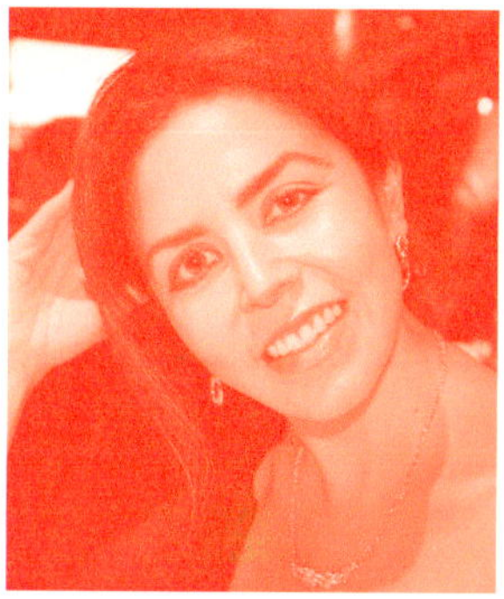

Supporting open minds since 2005

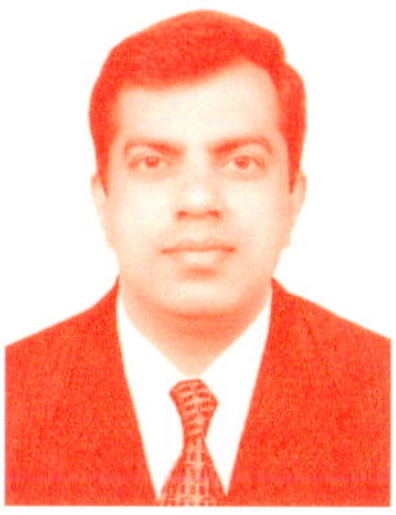

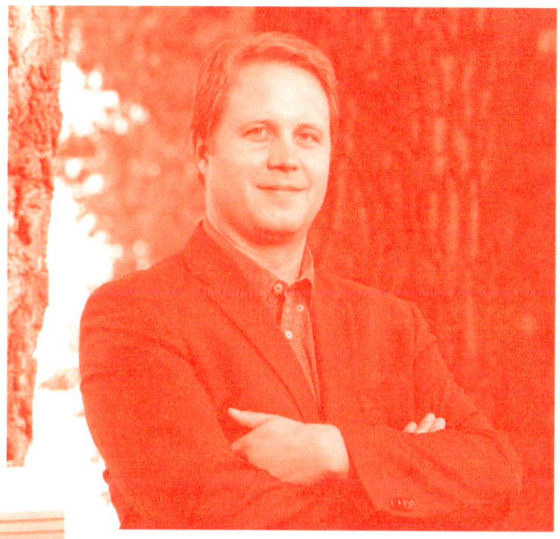

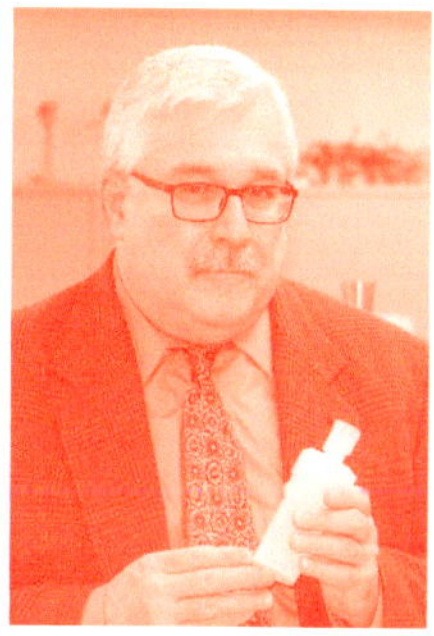

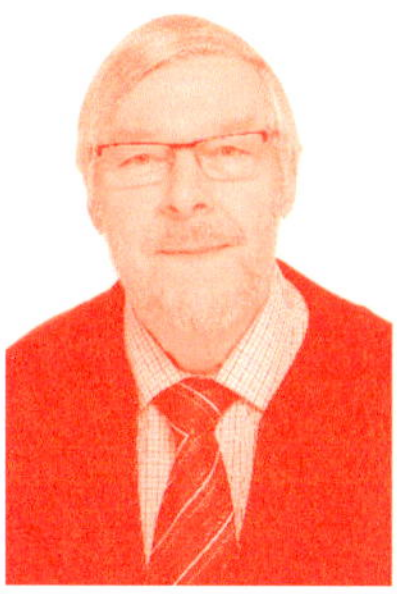

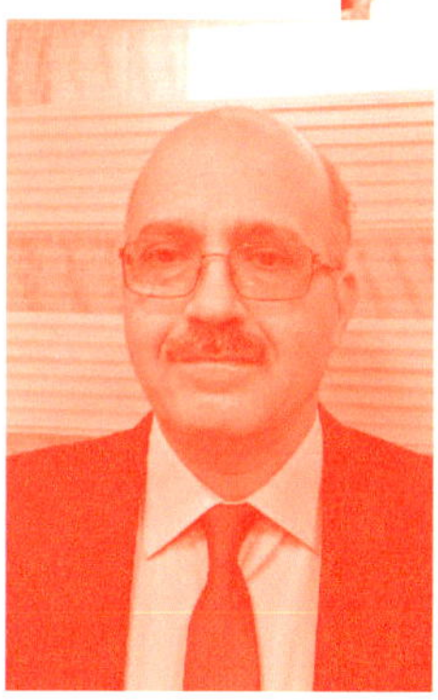

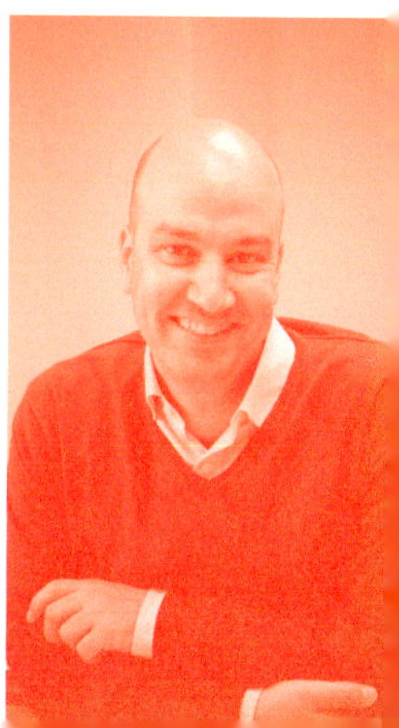

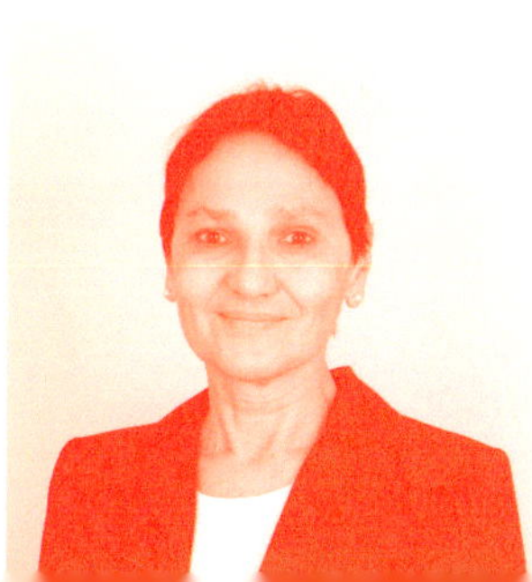

Connectivity and Functional Specialization in the Brain
http://dx.doi.org/10.5772/intechopen.87662
Edited by Thomas Heinbockel and Yongxia Zhou

Contributors
Heru Suwardianto, Umberto León-Domínguez, Yan M. Yufik, Rodrigo L. Castillo, Alejandro González-Candia, Nicole K. Rogers, Christian Xerri, Yoh'I Zennou-Azogui, Georgii Telegin, Aleksandr Chernov, Nikolay Konovalov, Alexey Belogurov, Irina Balmasova, Aleksandr Gabibov

First published in London, United Kingdom, 2021 by IntechOpen
IntechOpen is the global imprint of INTECHOPEN LIMITED, registered in England and Wales, registration number: 11086078, 5 Princes Gate Court, London, SW7 2QJ, United Kingdom
Printed in Croatia

British Library Cataloguing-in-Publication Data
A catalogue record for this book is available from the British Library

Additional hard and PDF copies can be obtained from orders@intechopen.com

Connectivity and Functional Specialization in the Brain
Edited by Thomas Heinbockel and Yongxia Zhou
p. cm.
Print ISBN 978-1-83962-796-5
Online ISBN 978-1-83962-797-2
eBook (PDF) ISBN 978-1-83962-798-9

For EU product safety concerns:
IN TECH d.o.o., Prolaz Marije Krucifikse Kozulić 3, 51000 Rijeka, Croatia, info@intechopen.com or visit our website at intechopen.com.

Meet the editors

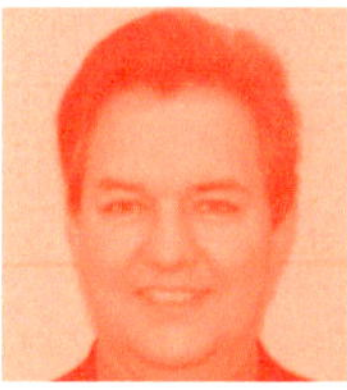

Thomas Heinbockel, Ph.D., is Professor and Interim Chair in the Department of Anatomy, Howard University College of Medicine, Washington, DC. Dr. Heinbockel's laboratory engages in multidisciplinary research to elucidate organizational principles of neural systems in the brain, specifically the limbic and olfactory systems. His research has been directed at understanding brain mechanisms of information processing and their relation to neurological and neuropsychiatric disorders. His lab works also on translational projects, specifically the development of novel anti-epileptic drugs and pharmacotherapeutic treatment options for drug addiction. His lab also analyzes drug actions at the epi- and genetic levels using next-generation sequencing technology. Dr. Heinbockel studied biology at the Philipps-University, Marburg, Germany. His studies of the brain began during his MS thesis work at the Max-Planck Institute for Behavioral Physiology, Starnberg/Seewiesen, Germany. Subsequently, Dr. Heinbockel completed a Ph.D. in Neuroscience at the University of Arizona, Tucson, Arizona, USA. After graduating, he was a research associate at the Institute of Physiology, Otto-von-Guericke-University School of Medicine, Magdeburg, Germany. Prior to his arrival at Howard University, Dr. Heinbockel held joint research faculty appointments in the Department of Anatomy and Neurobiology and the Department of Physiology at the University of Maryland School of Medicine, Baltimore, Maryland, USA. He still maintains an adjunct appointment in these departments.

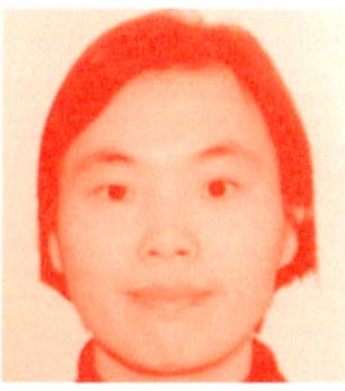

Yongxia Zhou obtained a Ph.D. in Biomedical Imaging from the University of Southern California. Her research interest is radiology and neuroscience technology and application. She had been trained as an imaging scientist at several prestigious institutes including Columbia University, the University of Pennsylvania, and the National Institutes of Health (NIH). Her research focuses on multi-modal neuroimaging integration such as MRI/PET and EEG/MEG instrumentation to make the best use of multiple modalities for better interpretation of underlying disease mechanisms. She is the author and editor of more than twelve books for well-known publishers including IntechOpen and Nova Science. She has published more than 100 papers and abstracts in many reputed international journals and conferences and served as reviewer and editor for several academic associations.

Contents

Preface

Neural connectivity is a topic that describes nerve cells in terms of their anatomical and functional connections. The term connectome refers to a comprehensive map of neural connections, like a wiring diagram of an organism's nervous system. Connectomics, the study of connectomes, can be applied to individual neurons and their synaptic connections, as well as to connections between neuronal populations or to functional and structural connectivity of different brain regions. This book, *Connectivity and Functional Specialization in the Brain*, addresses neural connectivity at these various scales in health and disease.

The chapters review novel findings related to neuroanatomy and cell biology, neurophysiology, neural plasticity, changes of connectivity in neurological disorders, and sensory system connectivity. The book provides the reader with an overview of the current state of the art of research of neural connectivity and focuses on the most important evidence-based developments in this area. Individual chapters focus on recent advances in specific areas of neural connectivity and in different brain regions. All chapters represent recent contributions to the rapidly developing field of neural connectivity.

The book is divided into two sections, each containing three chapters. Section 1 covers "Cellular and Clinical Aspects of Neural Connectivity" and Section 2 contains chapters on "Consciousness and Neural Connectivity".

Chapter One ("Cytokine Profile as a Marker of Cell Damage and Immune Dysfunction after Spinal Cord Injury"), written by G. Telegin, A. Chernov, N. Konovalov, A. Belogurov, I. Balmasova, and A. Gabibov, reviews experimental findings that investigate the role of key cytokines in the formation of a cellular response to trauma. In this case, trauma relates to spinal cord injury. The authors address the specific immunopathogenic interaction of the nervous and immune systems in the immediate and chronic post-traumatic periods.

In Chapter Two ("Blood–Brain Barrier Dysfunction in the Detrimental Brain Function"), Alejandro Gonzalez-Candia, Nicole K. Rogers, and Rodrigo L. Castillo debate the unique characteristics of the blood–brain barrier (BBB) as the interface of blood circulation and neural tissue. The authors discuss the existence of a neurovascular unit (NVU), which emphasizes that the dynamic BBB response to stressors requires coordinated interactions between various central nervous system cell types and structures. This chapter focuses on the structure and function of the BBB and how BBB breakdown causes detrimental brain function.

Chapter Three ("Physical and Cognitive Therapy (PCT) in Critically Ill Patient"), written by Heru Suwardianto, reviews the condition of critically ill patients in the Intensive Care Unit (ICU) who may have impaired physical and cognitive functions. The author aims to show that physical–cognitive therapy benefits physical and cognitive functions in critically ill patients in the ICU.

Chapter Four ("Brain Functional Architecture and Human Understanding"), written by Yan Yufik, addresses the basic question of what it means to understand and contrasts it with learning. The author focuses on different facets of understanding and formulates hypotheses regarding the underlying neuronal mechanisms, attempting to assess their plausibility and reconcile them with recent ideas and findings concerning brain functional architecture.

In Chapter Five ("The Neurofunctional Model of Consciousness: The Physiological Interconnectivity of Brain Networks"), Umberto Leon-Dominguez integrates neural networks' connectivity into a model that explores consciousness and volitional behavior from a neurofunctional perspective. The author proposes a theoretical evidenced-based framework that organizes brain pathways of neural information flow from the ascending reticular activating system and non-specific thalamic nuclei to cortical networks as functional neural loops. According to the author's model, the neural loops act as a global functional neural system, and their disruption due to brain damage can cause catastrophic outcomes, including cognitive and behavioral impairments.

In Chapter Six ("Interplay between Primary Cortical Areas and Crossmodal Plasticity"), Christian Xerri and Yoh'i Zennou-Azogui address a key concept of brain function, namely multisensory interaction and integration. The authors review the literature showing how multimodal interactions between primary cortices can contribute to refining perceptual representations. The authors also discuss how peripheral damage to a sensory system can result in multimodal integration to promote sensory substitution in deprived cortical areas and to favor compensatory plasticity in the spared sensory cortices.

We are grateful to IntechOpen for initiating this book project and for asking us to serve as its editors. Many thanks go to Marijana Francetic at IntechOpen for moving the project ahead in a timely fashion. Thanks are due to all contributors for taking the time to first write a chapter proposal, compose the chapter and, lastly, make our requested revisions to it. Hopefully, all contributors will continue their neural connectivity research with many intellectual challenges and exciting new directions. T.H. would like to thank his wife Dr. Vonnie D.C. Shields, Associate Dean and Professor, Towson University, Towson, MD, and their son Torben Heinbockel for the time that the editor was able to spend working on this book during the past year. Finally, T.H. is grateful to his parents Erich and Renate Heinbockel for their continuous support and interest in his work over many years.

Thomas Heinbockel, Ph.D.
Professor and Director of Graduate Studies,
Department of Anatomy,
Howard University College of Medicine,
Washington, DC, USA

Yongxia Zhou, Ph.D.
University of Southern California and Columbia University,
Los Angeles, California, USA

Section 1

Cellular and Clinical Aspects of Neural Connectivity

Chapter 1

Cytokine Profile as a Marker of Cell Damage and Immune Dysfunction after Spinal Cord Injury

Georgii Telegin, Aleksandr Chernov, Alexey Belogurov, Irina Balmasova, Nikolai Konovalov and Aleksandr Gabibov

Abstract

The study reviews findings of the recent experiments designed to investigate cytokine profile after a spinal cord injury. The role of key cytokines was assessed in the formation of cellular response to trauma. The specific immunopathogenic interaction of the nervous and immune systems in the immediate and chronic post-traumatic periods is summarized. The practicality of a step-by-step approach to assessing the cytokine profile in spinal cord injury is shown, the need to take into account the combination of pathogenetic and protective components in the implementation regulatory effects of individual cytokines, their integration into regenerative processes in the damaged spinal cord, which allows a rational approach to the organization of the treatment process and the development of new medicines.

Keywords: Spinal cord injury, glial scare, cytokines, cellular response

1. Introduction

Spinal cord injury (SCI) is a significant global public health issue and a common cause of permanent disability in patients [1, 2]. According to the WHO world population estimates, every year up to 500,000 people suffer a spinal cord injury [3], including young adults between the ages of 20 and 35 [4]. The annual incidence rate of traumatic SCI (TSCI) in developed countries is approx. 3 per 100,000 population [5], though these data could be inconsistent with the big picture, since 16%-30% of patients with spinal injuries die before being admitted to the hospital [6, 7]. Thus, functional recovery of the spinal cord with structural damages caused by trauma is recognized as one of the most challenging and socially essential topics of modern regenerative medicine [8].

Mortality from SCI depends mainly on the severity of spinal cord lesion, and at the pre-hospital phase, it reaches 37% [9]. In-hospital mortality rates are affected by the severity of spinal cord damage and the SCI-related early or late complications, as well as the timeliness of specialized health care provision. Mortality rates range between 8 and 58.3% in different medical settings, depending on their capacity [10–12]. High mortality rates (ranging between 16% and 18%) are reported for children. Frequently they are associated with a trauma of the cervical spine, especially its upper portion [13–16]. The leading causes of death comprise respiratory problems, cardiovascular disorders, thromboembolic events, infectious complications, and suicides [17]. Disability rates after vertebral column and spinal cord injuries vary from 57.5 to 100%, and the data indicate a trend towards an annual increase of people with disabilities after SCI [18].

Prominent underlying SCI causes include road traffic injuries (36–43%), falls from height (24.2–63.2%), shallow water diving (3–32%), sports activities and accidents (22.5%) [19–22], while criminal traumas account for 10-25% of the injuries [23]. The leading causes of injuries vary for different years and across geographic regions [24]. In this context, spinal cord injuries related to ocean waves are commonly reported in the coastal areas, among beachgoers, etc. [25].

Spinal cord injuries resulting from vertebral column trauma are reported for 36–72% of patients [10, 11, 26, 27]. Craniocerebral trauma is more commonly associated with cervical spine fractures (18–72%). Thoracic spine fractures are usually combined with multiple non-vertebral injuries, such as bone fractures (10.3–48%), traumas of the thoracic cavity and its internal organs (as high as 52%), and lumbar spine injuries – with broken limb bones (up to 27%) and pelvic bones (up to 15%), and damage of the abdominal organs (9.8–18.7%) [21, 27–31]. By type, SCIs are divided into open (penetrating) and closed (nonpenetrating) injuries to the spine. In peacetime, closed SCI account for 70.1–88.6% of cases [26, 32].

2. Factors that determine the course of spinal cord injury and its classification

The level and length of SCI, as well as the timeline of the treatment of spinal cord compression, affect the grade and severity of neurological problems and, ultimately, mobility and self-care of patients, as well as their prognosis and recovery, and return to normal life [33]. The cervical spine trauma is associated with spinal cord lesions in 12–70% of injured people and characterized by the predominance of severe damages (contusion, compression, haematomyelia) and high mortality rates (35–70%). Spinal cord lesions occur in 31–75% of thoracic and lumbar spine traumas [21, 26, 27, 29, 34]. In general, injuries of the cervical spine account for 17–61% of cases [30, 34], thoracic – 7.2–40% [26, 29, 34, 35], and lumbar spine – from 8.7 to 57.8% [26, 29, 31, 34].

Types of spinal cord trauma include contusion, concussion, compression, crush, and disruption. The spinal cord's compression is found in 20–26.7% of the injured persons, compression and contusion – in 40–50.5%, compression and crush – in 7–15.7%, and anatomical disruption – in 4.3–7.1% of patients [34]. The grade of the spinal cord injury is one of the principal prognostic factors. The distinction is made between "complete" and "incomplete" SCI, or its morphological disruption (anatomical or axonal). Complete SCI at the cervical level is reported for 33.7–52% of patients, thoracic level – 12.5-54%, and at the lumbar level – 15–21% [33].

In addition to SCI, non-traumatic spinal cord lesions may occur due to epidural abscess and hematoma, intradural tumor or other types of metastatic tumors, and complications after surgical treatment [7, 36]. The treatment of the acute phase in SCI cases takes more time than the treatment of spinal cord lesions of non-traumatic origin. Also, patients with SCI are more likely to have urinary tract infections and other complications [37].

Before early 1990s, a uniform or generally recognized classification system of SCI was not available. Physicians usually distinguished different levels of injury, complete and incomplete SCI.

Then, in 1992 the American Spinal Injury Association (ASIA) developed a classification system for identifying the severity of spinal cord injury based on descriptions of motor and sensory functions [38, 39].

1. A = complete spinal cord injury: no motor or sensory function is preserved in the sacral segments S4-S5;

2. B = incomplete injury: sensory function preserved but not motor function is preserved below the neurological level and includes the sacral segments S4-S5;

3. C = incomplete injury: motor function is preserved below the neurological level, but less than half of key muscles below the neurological level have a muscle grade less than 3 (i.e., they are not strong enough to move against gravity);

4. D = incomplete injury: motor function is preserved below the neurological level, and at least half of key muscles below the neurological level have a muscle grade of 3 or more (i.e., the joints can be moved against gravity);

5. E = normal: motor and sensory functions are normal.

Many researchers indicate that in addition to diagnostic implications the ASIA scale has tremendous prognostic value [38, 40–43]. Later, the AO Subaxial Cervical Spine Injury Classification (SLIC) system was published, which includes morphological information in its scoring that helps determine the extent of the patient's injury [44].

Practicing surgeons and radiologists use classification and scoring systems Subaxial Cervical Injury Classification and Severity (SLICS) and Thoracolumbar Injury Classification and Severity (TLICS), respectively, to evaluate the severity of cervical and thoracolumbar spine injuries [45]. Besides, the Spinal Cord Independence Measure (SCIM) has been developed to assess functional improvements of the spinal cord in the course of treatment and rehabilitation. Also, the SCIM has prognostic value [46].

SCI is classified chronologically into the following four phases:

1. acute phase – less than first 48 hours after the injury; the clinical course comprises of spinal shock and, as a result, the symptoms and signs are similar for various grades of SCI;

2. early (subacute) phase is defined to be 48 h – 14 days after the injury; likewise in the acute phase, clinical observations may include a syndrome of complete block of conduction in the spinal cord due to spinal shock, altered blood and cerebrospinal fluid flow; edema and swelling of the spinal cord;

3. intermediate phase is defined to be 14 days – 3 months; spinal shock symptoms disappear, and the actual severity and range of spinal cord injury is determined;

4. chronic phase – more than 3 months after the injury; the recovery of spinal cord functions occurs depending on the SCI grade; neurological status may deteriorate due to the scarring process, cyst formation, post-traumatic syringomyelia, etc. [23, 47–51].

Spinal cord injury triggers the development of a complex series of pathophysiological reactions, including primary and secondary damage of the nervous tissue [52–54]. The inflammatory response to the primary structural changes in the spinal cord is followed by the release of multiple regulatory peptides, including proinflammatory cytokines [55, 56].

3. A role of the immune system and cytokines in the acute phase of spinal cord injury

3.1 Cells of the nervous system in spinal cord injury as inductors, effectors and targets of inflammatory acute phase reactions

Two different phases are distinguished in the pathogenesis of the acute period of SCI; each of them is associated with a complex series of pathophysiological reactions in response to the nervous tissue damage [57, 58].

The first phase of the injury, which starts on the first day, immediately after mechanical trauma, involves mechanisms of the injury and disorders associated with these mechanisms. Neurons, astrocytes, oligodendrocytes, as well as other components of nerve signal transmission, are physically affected, and these events are accompanied by disorders of vascular components, including the blood–brain barrier (BBB) [56–60], which results in the tissue infiltration by inflammatory cells [61–63].

The inflammatory response to primary structural changes in the SC is associated with the release of multiple regulatory peptides, including proinflammatory ones, and cytokines [64, 65]. Cytokines are synthesized by the activated macro- and microglia, damaged vascular endothelium, as well as the immune system cells mobilized from the circulation system and transported to the site of injury and the adjacent areas due to a change in the BBB permeability [66].

It has been established that several important molecular components of the immune system, including tumor necrosis factor (TNF-α), inducible nitric oxide synthase (iNOS), nuclear factor (NF)-kB, interleukin (IL)-1β, and/or a factor of apoptosis Fas ligand (FasL), are activated as early as within a few minutes after SCI [67–69]. The activation of these molecules further results in inflammation and other kinds of significant neurological disorders [70].

The second phase comprises of endogenously induced degradation of the nervous tissue and associated consequences [70]. Increased glutamate concentration in the damaged spinal cord (SC) tissue induces neuronal excitotoxicity (a pathological process causing the neurotransmitter-mediated damage and death of nerve cells) due to the excess of intracellular Ca^{2+}. This process promotes the accumulation of reactive oxygen species [71–73], which, in turn, affect such cellular components as nucleic acids, proteins, and phospholipids and cause considerable cell losses and subsequent neurological dysfunction [74, 75].

It is important to highlight that the endogenous cells (neurons and glial cells) of human SC (but not the blood leukocytes) contribute to the early production of IL-1β, IL-6, and TNF-α during the post-traumatic inflammatory response [76–78].

Activated astrocytes represent the primary source of all damaging factors: they account for about 30% of the cellular composition; and the overexpression of the microRNA miR-136-5p in these cells during SCI is considered as one of the inducers of proinflammatory factors and chemokines (primarily TNF-α and IL-1β) [79–81]. This process triggers an inflammatory immune response involving type 17 T-helpers [82]. Angiogenesis mediated by microRNA (miR-210) is another SCI-related event [83, 84].

3.2 Distinct role of the innate immune cells and its cytokine release in acute phase reactions to spinal cord injury

However, the role of the immune cells secreting proinflammatory cytokines in SCI should not be underestimated. This process is stimulated by hemorrhages in the SC tissue after its damage [85, 86]. They contribute to the infiltration of affected regions by neutrophils, monocytes/macrophages, and T lymphocytes [87–90], i.e. cells releasing the same factors, i.e. TNF-α, IL-1α, IL-1β, and IL-6 [91, 92].

Typically, these cytokines reach their peak level 6–12 hours after the injury; they also induce an inflammatory response in acute and subacute phases and contribute to the lesion extension in rostral and caudal directions [93–95]. It was shown that activated microglia and macrophages infiltrating the SC are responsible for the subsequent necrosis and apoptosis of neurons, astrocytes, and oligodendrocytes located closely to the site of the lesion [96, 97], thus worsening the neurological outcome [98, 99]. The modulation of proinflammatory and immune effects in the SC tissue during its injury involves interferons through the increase in the number of stimulators of interferon genes (STING) in the tissue [100, 101].

Within the first 24 hours after SCI, an additional immunological effect takes place: the number of natural killer (NK) cells with an activated phenotype increases significantly, which is manifested by the overexpression of CD69, HLA-DR, NKG2D, and NKp30 on their membrane as well as the enhanced cytotoxic activity [102]. Furthermore, an increased level of the brain-derived neurotrophic factor (BDNF) that can be produced by vascular endothelial cells was found in the patients' plasma samples. At this phase of SCI, it strongly correlated with the percentage of NK cells and the expression of CD69 and NKp30 activating molecules on their surface [103].

Early interventions for reducing inflammation and preventing apoptosis have become a common strategy in the targeted medical care provided to SCI patients. However, the latest updates in this field suggest that the inflammatory process has apparent protective aspects that should not be ignored during treatment [104].

As for the cytokine release signals, they can enter the cells through the Toll-like receptors (TLRs) of the SC [105, 106]. TLRs are best known as the structures for pathogen recognition and initiation of the innate immune response [107, 108]. However, they can also detect tissue damage and trigger sterile inflammation by binding to endogenous ligands typical for stressed or damaged cells. In addition to the cells associated with the immune system, TLRs have also been identified in neurons of the central nervous system (CNS) and glial components, including microglia, astrocytes, and oligodendrocytes [109, 110]. To this end, Toll-like receptors may play both direct and indirect roles in SCI [111]. Indirect effects are most likely mediated by microglia or immune system cells penetrating the damaged CNS tissue [112]. It is also established that restorative responses in SCI-related ischemic disorders are taking place with the predominant participation of Toll-like receptor 3 and subsequent regulation by TLR4 [113].

One of the mechanisms of innate immune defense during SCI-related inflammatory response is associated with the unique role of mast cells [114]. Mast cells are abundant in the CNS and play an intricate role in the progression of neuroinflammatory disorders. In particular, it was shown that the experimental mast-cell deficient mice had increased astrogliosis and T-cell infiltration, while their functional recovery after SCI was significantly reduced [115]. Moreover, these mice have significantly increased levels of the cytokines MCP-1, NFα, IL-10, and IL-13 in the SC. The available data demonstrate the relationship between these findings and the fact that, if the same number and functional activity of mast cells are maintained, their chymases cleave MCP-1, IL-6, and IL-13. This suggests a protective role of the above cellular elements in the development of inflammatory changes in the nervous tissue in SCI cases [116]. It should be noted that, in addition to astrocytes and microglia, IL-10 is also produced by macrophages, B cells, and Th2 cells [117, 118]. Being an immunomodulator, IL-10 stimulates the generation of regulatory T cells while suppressing the activity of Th1 and NK cells [119].

The cytokine and hormone secretion pattern after spinal cord injury largely depends not only on the mechanisms of induction and immune response but also on the level of injury. Thus, the experiments in the rat model clearly demonstrated similar differences in the production of vascular endothelial growth factor (VEGF), leptin, interferon-γ-induced chemokine IP-10, IL-10, IL-18, granulocyte colony-stimulating factor (G-CSF), and chemokine fractalkine in animals' plasma. In contrast to the thoracic spine trauma, injury to the cervical spine is associated with a reduced expression of these mediators. A potential mechanism underlying this finding is sympathetic dysregulation caused by a higher location of the spine injury [120, 121]. Experiments in mice have also demonstrated that cytokines (e.g. interleukins IL-3, IL-6, IL-10, IL-13, and G-CSF) impacted the systemic changes after spinal cord injury in the lower thoracic region (Th910). In parallel, the activation of T lymphocytes and neutrophils was determined during the acute phase of the reported changes [122]. Thus, the immunopathogenic mechanisms primarily linked to innate immune cells and proinflammatory cytokines have a central role in the SCI acute phase.

Damaged neurons and neuroglial cells after spinal cord injury become a source of chemokines (fractalkine, MCP-1, and IP-10) [120, 122] targeting monocytes/macrophages and lymphocytes and promoting their entry into the lesion site. Mast cells represent one of the first cells of the innate immune system that exert their effect in the injury site. As already mentioned, mast cells can regulate chemokine secretion; however, their role is far from being clear. On the one hand, these cells can be a source of cytokines and other mediators promoting inflammation [123]. On the other hand, chymases released from mast cells during their activation and subsequent degranulation can destroy chemokines and proinflammatory cytokines, limiting the intensity of inflammatory response [116].

Most chemokines produced by cells of the injured spinal cord promote the recruitment of monocytes/macrophages [124], which eliminate cell debris, while chemokine IP-10 also recruits NK cells [125]. The involvement of NK cells in the innate immune response is also facilitated by the fact that after SCI the spinal cord cells express injury patterns, particularly stress-induced molecules (MICA, MICB), that are considered as ligands for NKG2D receptors [126]. In turn, their high level of expression by NK cells was demonstrated for spinal cord injury [101]. At first glance, manifestations of NK cells' cytotoxic activity against the nervous tissue in spinal cord injury significantly aggravate the destructive processes during trauma [101]. However, the involvement of NK cells in the elimination of exclusively the cells carrying injury patterns contributes to a more rapid suppression of destructive processes at the site of spinal cord lesion.

The study focused on another crucial player, macrophages, under the conditions of tissue damage has demonstrated that there are two stages of their activation [127]. During the first stage, these cells acquire an inflammatory (M1) phenotype mediated by endogenous molecules released during cellular damage. When reparative processes are triggered in response to damage at later stages, activated macrophages are polarized into the resident (M2) phenotype [127]. Thus, it is suggested that M1 macrophages are predominantly produced during the SCI acute phase. Their induction after SCI is also stimulated by interferons [128] that accumulate (as mentioned above) in the damaged tissues [100]. The macrophages secrete IL-12, IL-10, IL-1β, IL-6, IL-23, IL-21, TNF-α, and iNOS specific for this phenotype; high levels of these factors have been reported for the described pathological condition [120, 122, 127].

The cytokines have different functions: IL-12 further triggers adaptive cellular responses; IL-10 has an immunosuppressive effect and is involved in the induction of regulatory T cells; IL-1β, IL-6, IL-21, IL-23, and TNF-α exert a proinflammatory effect; TNF-α and iNOS provoke cellular damage reactions [128, 129].

The predominant cytokine profile, as well as the presence of M1 macrophage-producing cells in combination with the effect of autoantigens of the damaged spinal cord, suggests that the population of T lymphocytes involved in the immune response at the initial stage includes Th17 cells whose functional role has already been proven in the SCI acute phase. The functional role of this subpopulation is closely related to achieving the balance T-helper-17/regulatory T-cells (Th17/Treg). Q. Fu et al. [82] described these processes as follows. The Th17/Treg cell balance is regulated by molecules RORγT and FoxP3, while FoxP3 expression can be inhibited by RORγT expression. As mentioned above, SCI is accompanied by the migration of M1 macrophages to the injury site and the release of proinflammatory cytokines, including IL-6 and IL-21. As a result, T-helpers (CD^{4+} T lymphocytes) are able to differentiate into $CD^{4+}IL^{-}17A^{+}$ Th17, which contribute to the inflammatory response by recruiting neutrophilic granulocytes. In combination with proinflammatory cytokines produced at the injury site by macrophages, neurons, and neuroglia cells, the products of Th17 and neutrophils considerably enhance the inflammation process. Researchers consider the latter as a harmful component of the pathogenesis of post-traumatic changes in the spinal cord.

It is worth noting that Th17 induction during the initial phase requires one more cytokine, the transforming growth factor β (TGFβ), which is mainly secreted by Treg cells. The formation of these cells playing an important role in the Th17/Treg balance is mediated primarily by IL-10, which is also secreted by M1 macrophages in relatively small amounts during the initial phase of tissue damage. Like TGFβ, IL-10 has an immunosuppressive effect, limiting an excessive autoimmune inflammatory process after spinal cord injury [127, 130].

Thus, innate immune responses and T cell-mediated responses prevailing during the SCI acute phase could be assessed controversially. On the one hand, they aim to destroy cells in the damaged spinal cord tissue through their apoptosis or cytolysis and to induce inflammatory response enhancing neurological dysfunction. On the other hand, these reactions contribute to the elimination of destroyed cell elements along with their intrinsic autoantigens, injury patterns, and inflammation mediators, and also involve the inflammatory response regulation mechanisms. Based on these conclusions, a simplified approach cannot be used for assessing the role of immune processes in spinal cord injury. These processes are also important for selecting a treatment strategy during the SCI acute phase. It is necessary to evaluate the balance between the immune mechanisms prevailing in each particular case and exhibiting either a protective or pathogenic effect, instead of relying on individual indicators.

Already during the acute phase, spinal cord injury induces a strong inflammatory response [131] and a robust immune response both within and beyond the injury site [132]; these responses do not tend to resolve. In this case, the interaction takes place between the CNS and the immune system (i.e., the two central systems maintaining homeostasis in the entire body). That is why the process is not limited by the immune response in the site of spinal cord injury but also affects the whole immune system [133].

4. Role of the immune system and cytokines in the chronic phase of spinal cord injury

4.1 The importance of immunosuppressive manifestations in the chronic phase of spinal cord injury

The functions of the immune system change dramatically as the SCI acute phase progresses to the chronic stage. The failure or insufficient activity of vegetative innervation in the lymphatic and endocrine tissues disturb immune function for a long time after the initial trauma [134]. The main manifestations of such disorders are immune depression and the autoimmune process [133], although inflammatory reactions also maintain their significant role in pathogenesis.

Systemic changes at the level of cell populations and lymphocyte subpopulations during the SCI chronic phase are mainly related to the T cell-mediated adaptive immunity. Thus, it has been demonstrated that the total count of T cells (CD3+) and T helper cell subpopulation (CD3+ CD4+) in the blood is declining, although the count of activated CD4+ T cells (HLA-DR + CD4+) remains elevated [135]. This situation may occur if the count of T helper cells in the blood decreases due to their migration to the affected organ.

Regulatory T cells (Tregs) exhibiting suppressive properties are of special interest in this scenario. These cells have a CD3 + CD4 + CD25 + CD127lo phenotype with the predominance of activated CCR4 + HLA-Dr + fraction. The level of transforming growth factor β (TGFβ), the major cytokine of these cells, is considerably increased in SCI cases, which largely explains the observed immune dysfunction and its consequences, such as the impaired defense against infections and/or persistent chronic inflammation [88, 135].

The deficiency of T-cell-mediated immunity at the systemic level is also accompanied by a significant decrease in NK cell count during the chronic phase of SCI, which eventually leads to lethal infection [136].

Thus, starting on day 7 after the spinal cord injury, signs of regeneration of the myelin sheath of neurons associated with biochemically detectable activity of oligodendrocytes and production of proinflammatory cytokines TNF-α, IL-1β, and IL-6 were found [137]. Meanwhile, it was noted that a higher level of proinflammatory cytokines during the chronic phase correlated with a faster remission after SCI [51].

In fact, the proinflammatory cytokines trigger activation of astrocytes in the spinal cord glial tissue [138]. Astrocytes undergo proliferation and acquire one of the two phenotypes. Astrocytes having one phenotype actively secrete a glial fibrillary acidic protein (GFAP), which contributes to neuroregeneration. Contrariwise, astrocytes of the other phenotype secrete glutamine synthetase, which participates in glutamate accumulation and slows down neuronal regeneration in the injured spinal cord region. The balance between astrocytes of these two phenotypes determines the efficiency of repair processes in the neuronal tissue [139]. Neurons secrete neuregulin-1 (Nrg-1), which stimulates cell regeneration, contributes to the preservation of the spinal cord white matter, and positively regulates the functions of macrophages, T cells, and B cells. Today, it is even recommended as a medication for patients with spinal cord injury [140]. Although this positive regulation may occur, it is necessary to remember that all the described processes occur in the CNS; therefore, they can have both local and systemic manifestations.

Speaking about one of the key mechanisms of induction of the observed changes, a reference should be made to the data published by C.J. Ferrante and S.J. Leibovich [127]. They reported that after the acute phase of tissue damage, the macrophage phenotype switched abruptly from M1 to M2, which differs much from the typical M2 cells in terms of cytokine secretion. This variety was called the angiogenic M2d phenotype. The main products of M2d macrophage secretion included vascular endothelial growth factor (VEGF) and IL-10, inducing the formation of regulatory T cells. That is why the angiogenic and immunosuppressive effects are predominant. Similar transformations were also found for macrophage microglial cells [141].

Special focus is placed on the role of tumor necrosis factor α during the SCI chronic phase. During this phase, the level of brain-derived neurotrophic factor (BDNF) is decreasing in the hippocampus, and at the same time, it is rising in the lateral part of the spinal cord. A deletion within the gene encoding TNF-α receptor blocks this effect, but the presence of this cytokine restores the effect. These findings suggest that various structural synaptic changes in the spinal cord and hippocampal neurons are mediated by the overproduction of TNF-α in activated microglial cells, which can be associated with the development of chronic neuropathic pain and memory deficit after spinal cord injury [142]. IL-1β reducing the efficiency of calcium pump function in neurons also contributes to the development of neuropathic pain [143].

4.2 Autoimmune component of the chronic phase in spinal cord injury

Particular attention should be paid to the autoimmune processes associated with spinal cord injury. D.P. Ankeny et al. [144] demonstrated that spinal cord injury and related immunodepression cause profound long-lasting changes in the functions of B cells of the peripheral lymphoid tissue (the bone marrow and spleen) and the injured spinal cord. In particular, after their differentiation, the activated B cells are able to secrete autoantibodies that bind CNS proteins and nuclear antigens, including DNA and RNA. In patients with systemic lupus erythematosus, anti-DNA antibodies cross-reactively interact with glutamate receptors, causing excitotoxicity [145]. The same effect is reported for SCI-related autoantibodies, which exhibit similar neurotoxic properties.

After spinal cord injury, the autoimmunity can also promote CNS regeneration and/or neuroprotection, though a tendency towards neurotoxicity manifestations can still be present. Myelin-reactive T cells exhibit a similar neuroprotective effect in the rat model of SCI [146]. The data on the role played by autoantibodies are inconsistent. After all, the antibodies specific to CNS proteins can promote axonal regeneration and remyelination [147], as well as demyelination, because anti-myelin antibodies can participate in building a "bridge" between myelin of nerve fibers and oligodendrocytes [148]. In any case, despite the ambiguity of the effects and their interpretations, it has been verified that B cells infiltrate the injured spinal cord during the chronic phase [144].

The presented review demonstrates that the interpretation of the results is challenging because it is difficult to distinguish local and systemic effects after spinal cord injury. In this regard, the feasibility of differentiating between the local and systemic manifestations of immune response opens up certain prospects. For example, significant changes in the cytokine profile after SCI, especially during the chronic phase, were found not only in blood. Changes in the cytokine profile in CSF were even more informative. Thus, A.R. Taylor et al. [149] determined the levels of IL-2, IL-6, IL-7, IL-8, IL-10, IL-15, IL-18, granulocyte-macrophage colony-stimulating factor (GM-CSF), interferon-γ (IFNγ), keratinocyte chemoattractant (KC-like protein), IFNγ-inducible protein 10 (IP-10), monocyte chemotactic protein-1 (MCP-1), and tumor necrosis factor α (TNF-α) in cerebrospinal fluid as criteria characterizing the intensity of chronic inflammation. The concentrations of most cytokines and chemokines in CSF of animals after SCI correlated with the injury duration and trauma severity at sampling and the long-term neurological outcome. Thus, after spinal cord injury, the IL-8 level was significantly higher than in the control group of healthy animals but showed a negative correlation with the injury duration. At the same time, the levels of colony-stimulating factors and MCP-1 negatively correlated with the long-term positive outcome.

5. Conclusions

The review of publications focused on the problem of SCI-related immune (including cytokine) processes demonstrates that the available data are inconsistent and difficult to interpret.

Both the nervous and the immune systems have essential regulatory functions in the body and are tightly interrelated, while their interaction mechanisms are very diverse. Both local and systemic effects are associated with the neurological and immune changes occurring after spinal cord injury.

Along with these general aspects, the SCI-related local and systemic changes in the central nervous system and immune processes should be assessed on a stage-by-stage basis [150, 151]. Each phase is characterized by specific prevailing pathogenesis, which is initially linked to the response to injury and targeted at eliminating the damaged cells; then focus moves towards the inflammatory response with the aim of containing the affected area. Finally, a transition from local reactions to systemic processes occurs during later stages; the outcome of the pathological process depends on the efficiency of these phases. Each phase is associated with a specific category of immune response. In this respect, various cell subpopulations characterizing the innate and adaptive immunity or cytokines, the products secreted by these cells, can serve as markers of these immune responses [152, 153].

A specific feature of cytokines as markers of pathological changes after spinal cord injury is that they are secreted not only by immune cells but also by cells of the damaged spinal cord. The interaction between the nervous and immune systems can be characterized using the cytokine profile model. It has both theoretical research implications and diagnostic value and provides an opportunity to highlight the critical therapeutic targets.

Thus, cytokines contribute significantly to the pathogenesis of SCI-related traumatic disease and are responsible for its various manifestations. The cytokines can be secreted by immune cells; however, neurons of the damaged spinal cord are the main source of these biologically active substances. Therefore, the SCI-related cytokine pattern characterizes both the immune and neurological status and has a tremendous diagnostic and prognostic value.

Abbreviations

SC	spinal cord
SCI	spinal cord injury
CNS	central nervous system
BBB	blood–brain barrier

Author details

Georgii Telegin[1]*, Aleksandr Chernov[1], Alexey Belogurov[2], Irina Balmasova[3], Nikolai Konovalov[4] and Aleksandr Gabibov[2]

1 Branch of Shemyakin and Ovchinnikov Institute of Bioorganic Chemistry, Russian Academy of Sciences, Pushchino, Russia

2 Shemyakin and Ovchinnikov Institute of Bioorganic Chemistry, Russian Academy of Sciences, Moscow, Russia

3 Evdokimov Moscow State University of Medicine and Dentistry of Russia's Ministry of Health, Moscow, Russia

4 N.N. Burdenko National Scientific and Practical Center for Neurosurgery, Russian Federation Health Ministry, Moscow, Russia

*Address all correspondence to: telegin@bibch.ru

References

[1] Karsy M., Hawryluk G. Pharmacologic Management of Acute Spinal Cord Injury // Neurosurg Clin N Am. 2017. Vol. 28, № 1. P. 49-62.

[2] La Placa M.C., Simon C.M., Prado G.R., Cullen D.K. CNS injury biomechanics and experimental models // Prog Brain Res. 2007. Vol. 161. P. 13-26.

[3] Information bulleten WHO, № 384, November 2013.

[4] Braken M.B. Steroids for acute spinal cord injury // Cochrane Database Syst Rev. 2012. Vol. 1. CD001046.

[5] Safar P., Bicher N.D. Cardiopulmonary and cerebral resuscitation // M.: Medicine. 1997. 552 p.

[6] Leontiev M.A. Social adaptation of young disabled people with spinal cord injury by means of adaptive physical culture // Abstract of dissertation, Ph.D. Novokuzneck. 2003. 24 p.

[7] Sekhon L.H.S., Fehlings M.G. Epidemiology, demographics, and pathophysiology of acute spinal cord injury // Spine (Phila Pa 1976). 2001. Vol. 26. P. 2-12.

[8] Friedli L., Rosenzweig E.S., Barraud Q. et al. Pronounced species divergence in corticospinal tract reorganization and functional recovery after lateralized spinal cord injury favors primates // Sci Transl Med. 2015.- Vol. 7, №N 302. P. 134.

[9] Chipman J.G., Deuser W.E., Beilman G.J. Early surgery for thoracolumbar spine injuries decreases complications // J Trauma. 2004. Vol. 56, № l. P. 52-57.

[10] Gren' A.A. Surgical treatment of patients with spinal and spinal cord injuries with associated trauma // Abstract of dissertation, Ph.D. Moscow, 2008. 48 p.

[11] Orlov S.V., Shedrenko V.V., Mogychaya O.V. // Abstract science speech conference. Cheboksaru. 2006. P. 130-132.

[12] Bellet F.D., Rashid S.M., Jusabani M.A. et al. Traumatic Spine Injury: Which Discrepancy Between the Research Output and the Actual Burden of the Disease? // Pan Afr Med J. 2019. Vol. 33. P. 82.

[13] Nitecki S., Moir C.R. Predictive factors of the outcome of traumatic cervical spine fracture in children // J Pediatr Surg. 1994. Vol. 29, № 11. P. 1409-1411.

[14] Osenbach R.K., Menezes A.H. Pediatric spinal cord and vertebral column injury // Neurosurgery. 992. Vol. 30, № 3. P. 385-390.

[15] Eubanks J.D., Gilmore A., Bess S., Cooperman D.R. Clearing the pediatric cervical spine following injury // J Am Acad Orthop Surg. 2006. Vol. 14, № 9. p. 552-564.

[16] Poorman G.W., Segreto F.A., Beaubrun B.M. et al. Traumatic Fracture of the Pediatric Cervical Spine: Etiology, Epidemiology, Concurrent Injuries, and an Analysis of Perioperative Outcomes Using the Kids' Inpatient Database // Int J Spine Surg. 2019. Vol. 13, № 1. P. 68-78.

[17] Yeo J.D., Walsh J., Rutkowski S. et al. Mortality following spinal cord injury // Spinal Cord. 1998. Vol. 36. P. 329-336.

[18] Bogdanova L.P. A new complex of restorative treatment of patients with traumatic disease with complicated spine fractures // Abstract science speech conference. VI physiotherapeutic forum. SPb, 2006. P. 188.

[19] Kaikov A.K., Grin' A.A. TORACOSCOPIC SURGERY FOR INJURY OF THE CHEST SPINE // Grin' Tez. report All-Russian. scientific - practical. conf. "Polenov Readings". SPb. 2009. P. 89-90.

[20] Klimov V.S., Kostina E.V., Kireev D.O. Experience in treating patients with spinal cord injury in an emergency hospital // Abstract science speech conference VIII "Polenov Readings". SPb. 2009. P. 93.

[21] Mlavuxh S.G. Surgical tactics for unstable isolated and combined injuries of the thoracic and lumbar spine // Abstract of dissertation, Ph.D. M. 2009. 27 p.

[22] Gomes-Osman J., Cortes M., Guest J., Pascual-Leone A. A Systematic Review of Experimental Strategies Aimed at Improving Motor Function after Acute and Chronic Spinal Cord Injury // J Neurotrauma. 2016. Vol. 33, N 5. P. 425-438.

[23] Kanн S.L., Chyrlauev Yu.A. Intensive care for severe spinal cord injury // Politrauma. 2007. № 2. P. 65-75.

[24] H.-L. Li, H.Xu, Y.-L.Li et al. Epidemiology of traumatic spinal cord injury in Tianjin, China: An 18-year retrospective study of 735 cases // J Spinal Cord Med. 2019. Vol. 42, N 6. P. 778-785.

[25] Steinemann S., Galanis D.J., J.Cheng J. et al. Unique Epidemiology of Spinal Cord Injury in Hawai'i: Wave-related Incidents // Hawaii J Health Soc Welf. 2019. Vol. 78, №12. P. 365-370.

[26] Akshulakov S.K., Kerimbaev T.T. Epidemiology of spine and spinal cord injuries // Abstract science of conference neurosurgery Russia. SPb. 2002. P. 182.

[27] Alikov Z.U., Verhovskii A.I. Immediate results of surgical treatment of combined injuries of the thoracic and lumbar spine // Abstract science of conference «Surgery of spinal collum – full spectrum». M. 2007. P. 262-264.

[28] Voronovich I.R., Beleckii A.V., Dylyb O.I. et al. Diagnostics and treatment of traumatic polysegmental lesions of the spinal cord // Abstract science of conference «Surgery of spinal collum – full spectrum». M. 2007. P. 281-283.

[29] Dovlatov B.N., Maksudov B.M. Diagnostic algorithms and treatment tactics for multiple and concomitant spinal injuries // Abstract science of conference «Surgery of spinal collum – full spectrum». M. 2007. P. 288-289.

[30] Samoxvalov I.M., Badalov V.I., Korostulev K.E. et al. Treatment of severe concomitant spinal injuries // Tez. report All-Russian. scientific - practical. conf. "Polenov Readings". SPb. 2009. P. 99-100.

[31] Soloviev V.A., Telejkin V.V., Soloviev I.V. Our experience in the treatment of spinal injuries at the craniovertebral level // Tez. report All-Russian. scientific - practical. conf. Yioshkar-Ola. 2007. P. 83-85.

[32] Ball S.T., Vaccaro A.R., Albert T.J., Cotler J.M. Injuries of the thoracolumbar spine associated with restraint use in head-on motor vehicle accidents // Spinal Disorders. 2000. Vol. 13, N 4. P. 297-304.

[33] Morozov I.N., Mliavux S.G. Epidemiology of spine-spinal injury // Medical almanah (Niznii Novgorod). 2011. № 4 (17). 157-159.

[34] Perlmutter O.A. Compression of the spinal cord and its roots (diagnostics, surgical tactics) // Abstract of dissertation, Ph.D. M. 2000. 46 p.

[35] Dragun V.M. Surgical treatment of traumatic injuries of the middle

and lower cervical vertebrae // Traumatology and Orthopedics of Russia. 2008. № 3. P.82-83.

[36] Fassett D.R., Harrop J.S., Maltenfort M. et al. Mortality rates in geriatric patients with spinal cord injuries // J Neurosurg Spine. 2007. Vol. 7. P. 277-281.

[37] Gedde M.H., Lilleberg H.S., Abmus J. et al. Traumatic vs non-traumatic spinal cord injury: A comparison of primary rehabilitation outcomes and complications during hospitalization // J Spinal Cord Med. 2019. Vol. 42, N 6. P. 695-701.

[38] Vazquez X.M., Rodriguez M.S., Peñaranda J.M. et al. Determining prognosis after spinal cord injury // J Forensic Leg Med. 2008. Vol. 15, N 1. P. 20-23.

[39] Roberts T.T., Leonard G.R., Cepela D.J. Classifications in brief: American spinal injury association (ASIA) impairment scale // Clin Orthop Relat Res. 2017. Vol. 145, N 5. P. 1499-1504.

[40] Van Middendorp J.J., Hosman A.J., Donders A.R. et al. A clinical prediction rule for ambulation outcomes after traumatic spinal cord injury: a longitudinal cohort study // Lancet. - 2011. - Vol. 377, N 9770. P. 1004-1010.

[41] Van Middendorp J.J., Hosman A.J., Pouw M.H. et al. EM-SCI Study Group. ASIA impairment scale conversion in traumatic SCI: is it related with the ability to walk? A descriptive comparison with functional ambulation outcome measures in 273 patients // Spinal Cord. 2009. Vol. 47, N 7. P. 555-560.

[42] Van Middendorp J.J., Hosman A.J., Pouw M.H. et al. Is determination between complete and incomplete traumatic spinal cord injury clinically relevant? Validation of the ASIA sacral sparing criteria in a prospective cohort of 432 patients // Spinal Cord. 2009. Vol. 47, N 11. P. 809-816.

[43] Yarkony G., Chen D. Rehabilitation of patients with spinal cord injuries // In: R. Braddon (ed). Physical medicine and rehabilitation - W.B. Saunders Company. 1996. P. 1149-1179.

[44] H. Mushlin H., Kole M.J., Chryssikos T. et al. AOSpine Subaxial Cervical Spine Injury Classification System: The Relationship Between Injury Morphology, Admission Injury Severity, and Long-Term Neurologic Outcome // World Neurosurg. 2019. Vol. 130. P. 368-374.

[45] Perlmutter O.A. Spine and spinal cord injury // N. Novgorod. 2000. 144 p.

[46] Franceschini M., Bonavita J., Cecconi L. et al. Traumatic spinal cord injury in Italy 20 years later: current epidemiological trend and early predictors of rehabilitation outcome // Spinal Cord. 2020. 58(7):768-777.

[47] Berne J.D., Velmahos G.C., El-Tawil Q. et al. Value of complete cervical helical computed tomographic scanning in identifying cervical spine injury in the unevaluable blunt trauma patient with multiple injuries: a prospective study // J Trauma. 1999. Vol. 47. P. 896-902.

[48] Aimone J.B., Leasure J.L., Perreau V.M., Thallmair M. Spatial and temporal gene expression profiling of the contused rat spinal cord // Exp Neurol. 2004. Vol. 189, № 2. P. 204-221.

[49] Shechter R., Miller O., Yovel G. et al. Recruitment of Beneficial M2 Macrophages to Injured Spinal Cord Is Orchestrated by Remote Brain Choroid Plexus // Immunity. 2013. Vol. 38, N 3. P. 555-569.

[50] Chamankhah M., Eftekharpour E., Karimi-Abdolrezaee S. et al.

Genome-wide gene expression profiling of stress response in a spinal cord clip compression injury model // BMC Genomics. 2013. Vol. 14. P. 583-607.

[51] Moghaddam A., Child C., Bruckner T. et al. Posttraumatic Inflammation as a Key to Neuro-regeneration after Traumatic Spinal Cord Injury // Int J Mol Sci. 2015. Vol. 16, №4. P. 7900-7916.

[52] Marcol W., Slusarczyk W., Gzik M. et al. Air gun impactor--a novel model of graded white matter spinal cord injury in rodents // J Reconstr Microsurg. 2012. Vol. 28, № 8. P. 561-568.

[53] Oyinbo CA Secondary injury mechanisms in traumatic spinal cord injury: a nugget of this multiply cascade // Acta Neurobiol Exp (Wars). 2011;71(2):281-99.

[54] Ren H., Chen X., Tian M. et al. Regulation of Inflammatory Cytokines for Spinal Cord Injury Repair Through Local Delivery of Therapeutic Agents // Adv. Sci. 2018, 5, 1800529.

[55] Zhang N., Yin Y., Xu S.J. et al. Inflammation and apoptosis in spinal cord injury // Indian J Med Res. 2012, 135 (3); 287-296.

[56] Cruz C. D., Coelho A., Antunes-Lopes T., Cruz F. Biomarkers of spinal cord injury and ensuing bladder dysfunction // Adv. Drug Delivery Rev. 2015, 82-83, 153.

[57] Gruys E, Toussaint MJ, Niewold TA, Koopmans SJ. Acute phase reaction and acute phase proteins // J Zhejiang Univ Sci B. 2005;6(11):1045-1056. doi:10.1631/jzus.2005.B1045.

[58] Zhang N., Yin Y., Xu S.J., Wu Y.P., Chen W.S. Inflammation & apoptosis in spinal cord injury // Indian J. Med. Res. 2012. V. 135. № 3. P. 287-296.

[59] Wilcox J.T., Satkunendrarajah K., Nasirzadeh Y., et. al Generating level-dependent models of cervical and thoracic spinal cord injury: Exploring the interplay of neuroanatomy, physiology, and function.// Neurobiol. Dis. 2017. V. 105. P. 194-212.

[60] Figley S.A., Khosravi R., Legasto J.M., Tseng Y.-F., Fehlings M.G. Characterization of vascular disruption and blood-spinal cord barrier permeability following traumatic spinal cord injury // J. Neurotrauma. 2014. V. 31. № 6. P. 541-552.

[61] Kunis G., Baruch K., Rosenzweig N., Kertser A., Miller O., Berkutzki T., Schwartz M. IFN-γ-dependent activation of the brain's choroid plexus for CNS immune surveillance and repair // Brain. 2013. V. 136. № 11. P. 3427-3440.

[62] Li Y., Lucas-Osma A.M., Black S., Bandet M.V., Stephens M.J., Vavrek R., Sanelli L., Fenrich K.K., Di Narzo A.F., Dracheva S., et al. Pericytes impair capillary blood flow and motor function after chronic spinal cord injury // Nat. Med. 2017. V. 23. № 6. P. 733-741.

[63] Shechter R., Miller O., Yovel O.G., Rosenzweig N., London A., Ruckh J., Kim K.-W., Klein E., Kalchenko V., Bendel P., et al. Recruitment of beneficial M2 macrophages to injured spinal cord is orchestrated by remote brain choroid plexus // Immunity. 2013. V. 38. № 3. P. 555-569.

[64] Goss J.R., Taffe K.M., Kochanek P.M., DeKosky S.T. The antioxidant enzymes glutathione peroxidase and catalase increase following traumatic brain injury in the rat // Exp. Neurol. 1997. V. 146. № 1. P. 291-294.

[65] Ren H., Chen X., Tian M., Zhou J., Ouyang H., Zhang Z. Regulation of Inflammatory Cytokines for Spinal Cord Injury Repair Through Local Delivery of Therapeutic Agents // Adv. Sci. 2018. V. 5. № 11. P. 1800529.

[66] Sutherland TC, Mathews KJ, Mao Y, Nguyen T, Gorrie CA. Differences in the Cellular Response to Acute Spinal Cord Injury between Developing and Mature Rats Highlights the Potential Significance of the Inflammatory Response // Front. Cell Neurosci. 2017. V. 10. P. 310.

[67] Shohami E., Bass R., Wallach D., Yamin A., Gallily R. Inhibition of tumor necrosis factor alpha (TNFalpha) activity in rat brain is associated with cerebroprotection after closed head injury // J. Cereb. Blood Metabol. 1996. V. 16. № 3. P. 378-384.

[68] Yu W.R., Fehlings M.G. Fas/FasL-mediated apoptosis and inflammation are key features of acute human spinal cord injury: implications for translational, clinical application // Acta Neuropathol. 2011. V. 122. № 6. P. 747-761.

[69] Chen S., Ye J., Chen X., Shi J., Wu W., Lin W., Lin W., Li Y., Fu H., Li S. Valproic acid attenuates traumatic spinal cord injury-induced inflammation via STAT1 and NF-κB pathway dependent of HDAC3 // J. Neuroinflammation. 2018. V. 15. № 1. P. 150-163.

[70] Jorge A., Taylor T., Agarwal N., Hamilton D.K. Current agents and related therapeutic targets for inflammation after acute traumatic spinal cord injury // World Neurosurg. 2019. V. 132. P. 138-147.

[71] Breckwoldt M.O., Pfister F.M., Bradley P.M., Marinković P., Williams P.R., Brill M.S., Plomer B., Schmalz A., St Clair D.K., Naumann R., et al. Multiparametric optical analysis of mitochondrial redox signals during neuronal physiology and pathology in vivo // Nat. Med. 2014. V. 20. № 5. P. 555-560.

[72] Ouardouz M., Coderre E., Basak A., Chen A., Zamponi G.W., Hameed S., Rehak R., Yin X., Trapp B.D., Stys P.K. Glutamate receptors on myelinated spinal cord axons: I. GluR6 kainate receptors // Ann. Neurol. 2009. V. 65. № 2. P. 151-159.

[73] Yin H.Z., Hsu C.I., Yu S., Rao S.D., Sorkin L.S., Weiss J.H. TNF-α triggers rapid membrane insertion of Ca2+ permeable AMPA receptors into adult motor neurons and enhances their susceptibility to slow excitotoxic injury // Exp. Neurol. 2012. V. 238. № 2. P. 93-102.

[74] Khayrullina G., Bermudez S., Byrnes K.R. Inhibition of NOX2 reduces locomotor impairment, inflammation, and oxidative stress after spinal cord injury // J. Neuroinflammation. 2015. V. 12. P. 172-182.

[75] Von Leden R.E., Khayrullina G., Moritz K.E., Byrnes K.R. Age exacerbates microglial activation, oxidative stress, inflammatory and NOX2 gene expression, and delays functional recovery in a middle-aged rodent model of spinal cord injury // J. Neuroinflammation. 2017. V. 14. № 1. P. 161-174.

[76] Pineau I., Lacroix S. Proinflammatory cytokine synthesis in the injured mouse spinal cord: multiphasic expression pattern and identification of the cell types involved // J. Comp. Neurol. 2007. V. 500. № 2. P. 267-285.

[77] Yang L., Blumbergs P.C., Jones N.R., Manavis J., Sarvestani G.T., Ghabriel M.N. Early expression and cellular localization of proinflammatory cytokines interleukin-1beta, interleukin-6, and tumor necrosis factor-alpha in human traumatic spinal cord injury // Spine. 2004. V. 29. № 9. P. 966-971.

[78] Yang L., Jones N.R., Blumbergs P.C., van den Heuvel C., Moore E.J., Manavis J., Sarvestani G.T., Ghabriel M.N. Severity-dependent

expression of pro-inflammatory cytokines in traumatic spinal cord injury in the rat // J. Clin. Neurosci. 2005. V. 12. № 3. P. 276-284.

[79] Deng G., Gao Y., Cen Z., He J., Cao B., Zeng G., Zong S. miR-136-5p Regulates the Inflammatory Response by Targeting the IKKβ/NF-κB/A20 Pathway After Spinal Cord Injury // Cell Biochem. 2018. V. 50. № 2. P. 512-524.

[80] He J., Zhao J., Peng X., Shi X., Zong S., Zeng G. Molecular Mechanism of MiR-136-5p Targeting NF-κB/A20 in the IL-17-Mediated Inflammatory Response after Spinal Cord Injury // Cell Physiol. Biochem. 2017. V. 44. № 3. P. 1224-1241.

[81] Beilerli O.A., Azizova Sh.T., Konovalov N.A., Akhmedov A.D., Gareev I.F., Belogurov A.A. Non-coding rna as therapeutic targets for spinal cord injury // Questions of neurosurgery named after N.N. Burdenko . 2020. Vol. 84. № 4. P. 104-110.

[82] Fu Q., Liu Y., Liu X., Zhang Q., Chen L., Peng J., Ao J., Li Y., Wang S., Song G., et al. Engrafted peripheral blood-derived mesenchymal stem cells promote locomotive recovery in adult rats after spinal cord injury // Am. J. Transl. Res. 2017. V. 9. № 9. P. 3950-3966.

[83] Cao Y., Wu T.D., Wu H., Lang Y., Li D.Z., Ni S.F., Lu H.B., Hu J.Z. Synchrotron radiation micro-CT as a novel tool to evaluate the effect of agomir-210 in a rat spinal cord injury model // Brain Res. 2017. V. 1655. P. 55-65.

[84] Ujigo S., Kamei N., Hadoush H., FujiokaY., MiyakiS., NakasaT., TanakaN., Nakanishi K., Eguchi A., Sunagawa T., et al. Administration of microRNA-210 promotes spinal cord regeneration in mice // Spine. 2014. V. 39. № 14. P. 1099-1107.

[85] Saiwai H., Ohkawa Y., Yamada H., Kumamaru H., Harada A., Okano H., Yokomizo T., Iwamoto Y., Okada S. The LTB4-BLT1 axis mediates neutrophil infiltration and secondary injury in experimental spinal cord injury // Am. J. Pathol. 2010. V. 176. № 5. P. 2352-2366.

[86] Yokota K., Saito T., Kobayakawa K., Kubota K., Hara M., Murata M., Ohkawa Y., Iwamoto Y., Okada S. The feasibility of in vivo imaging of infiltrating blood cells for predicting the functional prognosis after spinal cord injury // Sci. Rep. 2016. V. 6. P. 25673-25684.

[87] Ankeny D.P., Guan Z., Popovich P.G. B cells produce pathogenic antibodies and impair recovery after spinal cord injury in mice // J. Clin. Invest. 2009. V. 119. № 10. P. 2990-2999.

[88] Beck K.D., Nguyen H.X., Galvan M.D., Salazar D.L., Woodruff T.M., Anderson A.J. Quantitative analysis of cellular inflammation after traumatic spinal cord injury: evidence for a multiphasic inflammatory response in the acute to chronic environment // Brain. 2010. V. 133. Pt. 2. P. 433-447.

[89] Raposo C., Graubardt N., Cohen M., Eitan C., London A., Berkutzki T., Schwartz M. CNS repair requires both effector and regulatory T cells with distinct temporal and spatial profiles // J. Neurosci. 2014. V. 34. № 31. P. 10141-10155.

[90] Saiwai H., Kumamaru H., Ohkawa Y., Kubota K., Kobayakawa K., Yamada H., Yokomizo T., Iwamoto Y., Okada S. // J. Neurochem. 2013. V. 125. № 1. P. 74-88.

[91] Kumamaru H., Saiwai H., Ohkawa Y., Yamada H., Iwamoto Y., Okada S., Ly6C+ Ly6GMyeloid-derived suppressor cells play a critical role in the resolution of acute inflammation and the subsequent tissue repair process after spinal cord injury // J. Cell Physiol. 2012. V. 227. № 4. P. 1335-1346.

[92] Nguyen D.H., Cho N., Satkunendrarajah K., Austin J.W., Wang J., Fehlings M.G. Immunoglobulin G (IgG) attenuates neuroinflammation and improves neurobehavioral recovery after cervical spinal cord injury // J. Neuroinflammation. 2012. V. 9. P. 224-237.

[93] Min K.J., Jeong H.K., Kim B., Hwang D.H., Shin H.Y., Nguyen A.T., Kim J.H., Jou I., Kim B.G., Joe E.H. Spatial and temporal correlation in progressive degeneration of neurons and astrocytes in contusion-induced spinal cord injury // J. Neuroinflammation. 2012. V. 9. P. 100-112.

[94] Smith P.D., Puskas F., Meng X., Lee J.H., Cleveland J.C. Jr., Weyant M.J., Fullerton D.A., Reece T.B. The evolution of chemokine release supports a bimodal mechanism of spinal cord ischemia and reperfusion injury // Circulation. 2012. V. 126. № 11(1). P. 110-117.

[95] Zhu P., Li J.X., Fujino M., Zhuang J., Li X.K. Development and treatments of inflammatory cells and cytokines in spinal cord ischemia-reperfusion injury // Mediators Inflamm. 2013. V. 2013. P. 701970.

[96] Akhmetzyanova E., Kletenkov K., Mukhamedshina Y., Rizvanov A. Different Approaches to Modulation of Microglia Phenotypes After Spinal Cord Injury // Front. Syst. Neurosci. 2019. V. 13. P. 37-48.

[97] Chu G.K., Yu W., Fehlings M.G. The p75 neurotrophin receptor is essential for neuronal cell survival and improvement of functional recovery after spinal cord injury // Neuroscience. 2007. V. 148. № 3. P. 668-682.

[98] Floriddia E.M., Rathore K.I., Tedeschi A., Quadrato G., Wuttke A., Lueckmann J.M., Kigerl K.A., Popovich P.G., Di Giovanni S. p53 Regulates the neuronal intrinsic and extrinsic responses affecting the recovery of motor function following spinal cord injury // J. Neurosci. 2012. V. 32. № 40. P. 13956-13970.

[99] Horn K.P., Busch S.A., Hawthorne A.L., van Rooijen N., Silver J. Another barrier to regeneration in the CNS: activated macrophages induce extensive retraction of dystrophic axons through direct physical interactions // J. Neurosci. 2008. V. 28. № 38. P. 9330-9341.

[100] Roselli F., Chandrasekar A., Morganti-Kossmann M.C. Interferons in Traumatic Brain and Spinal Cord Injury: Current Evidence for Translational Application // Front. Neurol. 2018. V. 9. P. 458.

[101] Wang Y.Y., Shen D., Zhao L.J., Zeng N., Hu T.H. Sting is a critical regulator of spinal cord injury by regulating microglial inflammation via interacting with TBK1 in mice // Biochem. Biophys. Res. Commun. 2019. V. 517. № 4. P. 741-748.

[102] Laginha I., Kopp M.A., Druschel C., Schaser K.D., Brommer B., Hellmann R.C., Watzlawick R., Ossami-Saidi R.R., Prüss H., Failli V., et al Natural Killer (NK) Cell Functionality after human Spinal Cord Injury (SCI): protocol of a prospective, longitudinal study // BMC Neurol. 2016. V. 16. № 1. P. 170.

[103] Xu L., Zhang Y., Zhang R., Zhang H., Song P., Ma T., Li Y., Wang X., Hou X., Li Q., et al. Elevated plasma BDNF levels are correlated with NK cell activation in patients with traumatic spinal cord injury // Int. Immunopharmacol. 2019. V. 74. P. 105722.

[104] Rust R., Kaiser J. Insights into the Dual Role of Inflammation after Spinal Cord Injury // J. Neurosci. 2017. V. 37. № 18. P. 4658-4660.

[105] Azam S., Jakaria M., Kim I.S., Kim J., Haque M.E., Choi D.K. Regulation of Toll-Like Receptor (TLR) Signaling Pathway by Polyphenols in the Treatment of Age-Linked Neurodegenerative Diseases: Focus on TLR4 Signaling // Front. Immunol. 2019. V. 10. P. 1000.

[106] Kigerl K.A., Popovich P.G. Toll-like receptors in spinal cord injury // Curr. Top Microbiol. Immunol. 2009. V. 336. P. 121-136.

[107] Hug H., Mohajeri M.H., La Fata G. Toll-Like Receptors: Regulators of the Immune Response in the Human Gut // Nutrients. 2018. V. 10. № 2. P. 203.

[108] Kawasaki T., Kawai T. Toll-like receptor signaling pathways // Front. Immunol. 2014. V. 5. P. 461.

[109] Marinelli C., Di Liddo R., Facci L., Bertalot T., Conconi M.T., Zusso M., Skaper S.D., Giusti P. Ligand engagement of Toll-like receptors regulates their expression in cortical microglia and astrocytes / J. Neuroinflammation. 2015. V. 12. P. 244.

[110] Trudler D., Farfara D., Frenkel D. Toll-like receptors expression and signaling in glia cells in neuro-amyloidogenic diseases: towards future therapeutic application / Mediators Inflamm. 2010. V. 2010. P. 497987.

[111] Lacagnina M.J., Watkins L.R., Grace P.M. Toll-like receptors and their role in persistent pain // Pharmacol. Ther. 2018. V. 184. P. 145-158.

[112] Heiman A., Pallottie A., Heary R.F., Elkabes S. Toll-like receptors in central nervous system injury and disease: a focus on the spinal cord // Brain Behav. Immun. 2014. V. 42. P. 232-245.

[113] Lobenwein D., Tepekoylu C., Kozarin R. et al. Shock Wave Treatment Protects From Neuronal Degeneration via a Toll-Like Receptor 3 Dependent Mechanism: Implications of a First-Ever Causal Treatment for Ischemic Spinal Cord Injury // J. Am. Heart. Assoc. 2015. V. 4. № 10. e002440.

[114] Mittal A., Sagi V., Gupta M., Gupta K. Mast Cell Neural Interactions in Health and Disease // Front. Cell Neurosci. 2019. V. 13. P. 110-115.

[115] Vangansewinkel T., Geurts N., Quanten K., Nelissen S., Lemmens S., Geboes L., Dooley D., Vidal P.M., Pejler G., Hendrix S. Mast cells promote scar remodeling and functional recovery after spinal cord injury via mouse mast cell protease 6 // FASEB J. 2016. V. 30. № 5. P. 2040-2057.

[116] Nelissen S., Vangansewinkel T., Geurts N., Geboes L., Lemmens E., Vidal P.M., Lemmens S., Willems L., Boato F., Dooley D., et al. Mast cells protect from post-traumatic spinal cord damage in mice by degrading inflammation-associated cytokines via mouse mast cell protease 4 // Neurobiol. Dis. 2014. V. 62. P. 260-272.

[117] Rutz S., Ouyang W. Regulation of Interleukin-10 Expression // Adv. Exp. Med. Biol. 2016. V. 941. P. 89-116.

[118] Rutz S., Ouyang W. Regulation of interleukin-10 and interleukin-22 expression in T helper cells // Curr. Opin. Immunol. 2011. V. 23. № 5. P. 605-612.

[119] Lobo-Silva D., Carriche G.M., Castro A.G., Roque S., Saraiva M. Balancing the immune response in the brain: IL-10 and its regulation // J. Neuroinflammation. 2016. V. 13. № 1. P. 297.

[120] Hong J., Chang A., Zavvarian M.M., Wang J., Liu Y., Fehlings M.G. Level-Specific Differences in Systemic Expression of Pro- and Anti-Inflammatory Cytokines and Chemokines after Spinal Cord Injury // Int. J. Mol. Sci. 2018. V. 19. № 8. P. 2167-2178.

[121] Hong J., Chang A., Liu Y., Wang J., Fehlings M.G. Incomplete Spinal Cord Injury Reverses the Level-Dependence of Spinal Cord Injury Immune Deficiency Syndrome // Int. J. Mol. Sci. 2019. V. 20. № 15. P. 3762.

[122] Yuan X., Wu Q., Tang Y., Jing Y., Li Z., Xiu R. Systemic microcirculation dysfunction after low thoracic spinal cord injury in mice // Life Sci. 2019. V. 221. P. 47-55.

[123] Tsibulkina V.N., Tsibulkin N.A. Mast cell as a polyfunctional element of the immune system // Allergology and immunology in pediatrics. 2017. Vol. 2. P. 4-11.

[124] Sarbaeva N.N., Ponomareva Yu.V., Milyakova M.N. Macrophages: variety of phenotypes and functions, interaction with foreign materials // Genes and cells. 2016. Vol. XI. № 1. P. 9-17.

[125] Zhang Y., Gao Z., Wang D., Zhang T., Sun B., Mu L., Wang J., Liu Y., Kong Q., Liu X., et al. Accumulation of natural killer cells in ischemic brain tissues and the chemotactic effect of IP-10 // J. Neuroinflammation. 2014. V. 11. P. 79.

[126] Balmasova I.P., Shmeleva E.V., Eremina O.F., Dunda N.I. Characteristics of the regulatory-receptor apparatus of natural killer cells in clinically healthy people q // Allergology and immunology. 2009. Vol. 10. № 2. P. 169.

[127] Ferrante C.J., Leibovich S.J. Regulation of Macrophage Polarization and Wound Healing // Adv. Wound Care (New Rochelle). 2012. V. 1. № 1. P. 10-16.

[128] Balmasova I.P., Nesterova I.V., Malova E.S., Sepiashvili R.I. Structural and functional organization of the immune system. Moscow: Practical Medicine, 2019. 72 p.

[129] Chubenko V.A. Immunotherapy based on cytokines (Il-1. Il-2. Tnf. Ksf. Interferons) // Practical oncology. 2016. T. 17. № 2. C. 99-109.

[130] Fasching P., Stradner M., Graninger W., Dejaco C., Fessler J. Therapeutic Potential of Targeting the Th17/Treg Axis in Autoimmune Disorders // Molecules. 2017. V. 22. № 1. P. 134.

[131] Rice T., Larsen J., Rivest S., Yong V.W. Characterization of the early neuroinflammation after spinal cord injury in mice // J. Neuropathol. Exp. Neurol. 2007. V. 66. № 3. P. 184-195.

[132] Irwin M.R., Cole S.W. Reciprocal regulation of the neural and innate immune systems // Nat. Rev. Immunol. 2011. V. 11. № 9. P. 625-632.

[133] Schwab J.M., Zhang Y., Kopp M.A., Brommer B., Popovich P.G. The paradox of chronic neuroinflammation, systemic immune suppression, autoimmunity after traumatic chronic spinal cord injury // Exp. Neurol. 2014. V. 258. P. 121-129.

[134] Zhou Y., Li N., Zhu L., Lin Y., Cheng H. The microglial activation profile and associated factors after experimental spinal cord injury in rats // Neuropsychiatr. Dis Treat. 2018. V. 14. P. 2401-2413.

[135] Monahan R., Stein A., Gibbs K., Bank M., Bloom O. Circulating T cell subsets are altered in individuals with chronic spinal cord injury // Immunol. Res. 2015. V. 63. № 1-3. P. 3-10.

[136] Herman P., Stein A., Gibbs K., Korsunsky I., Gregersen P., Bloom O. Persons with Chronic Spinal Cord Injury Have Decreased Natural Killer Cell and Increased Toll-Like Receptor/ Inflammatory Gene Expression // J. Neurotrauma. 2018. V. 35. № 15. P. 1819-1829.

[137] Zhang Y., Guan Z., Reader B., Shawler T., Mandrekar-Colucci S., Huang K., Weil Z., Bratasz A., Wells J., Powell N.D., et al. Autonomic dysreflexia causes chronic immune suppression after spinal cord injury // J. Neurosci. 2013. V. 33. № 32. P. 12970-12981.

[138] Sanz P., Garcia-Gimeno M.A. Reactive Glia Inflammatory Signaling Pathways and Epilepsy // Int. J. Mol. Sci. 2020. V. 21. № 11. P. 4096-4112.

[139] Pekny M., Pekna M. Astrocyte reactivity and reactive astrogliosis: costs and benefits // Physiol. Rev. 2014. V. 94. № 4. P. 1077-1098.

[140] Alizadeh A., Santhosh K.T., Kataria H., Gounni A.S., Karimi-Abdolrezaee S. Neuregulin-1 elicits a regulatory immune response following traumatic spinal cord injury // J. Neuroinflammation. 2018. V. 15. № 1. P. 53-73.

[141] Gensel J.C., Zhang B. Macrophage activation and its role in repair and pathology after spinal cord injury // Brain Res. 2015. V. 1619. P. 1-11.

[142] Liu Y., Zhou L.J., Wang J., Li D., Ren W.J., Peng J., Wei X., Xu T., Xin W.J., Pang R.P., et al. TNF-α Differentially Regulates Synaptic Plasticity in the Hippocampus and Spinal Cord by Microglia-Dependent Mechanisms after Peripheral Nerve Injury// J. Neurosci. 2017. V. 37. № 4. P. 871-881.

[143] Mirabelli E., Ni L., Li L., Acioglu C., Heary R.F., Elkabes S. Pathological pain processing in mouse models of multiple sclerosis and spinal cord injury: contribution of plasma membrane calcium ATPase 2 (PMCA2) // J. Neuroinflammation. 2019. V. 16. № 1. P. 207.

[144] Ankeny D.P., Lucin K.M., Sanders V.M., McGaughy V.M., Popovich P.G. Spinal cord injury triggers systemic autoimmunity: evidence for chronic B lymphocyte activation and lupus-like autoantibody synthesis // J. Neurochem. 2006. V. 99. P. 1073-1087.

[145] DeGiorgio L.A., Konstantinov K.N., Lee S.C., Hardin J.A., Volpe B.T., Diamond B. A subset of lupus anti-DNA antibodies cross-reacts with the NR2 glutamate receptor in systemic lupus erythematosus // Nat. Med. 2001. V. 7. № 11. P. 1189-1193.

[146] Hauben E., Butovsky O., Nevo U., Yoles E., Moalem G., Agranov E., Mor F., Leibowitz-Amit R., Pevsner E., Akselrod S., et al. Passive or Active Immunization with Myelin Basic Protein Promotes Recovery from Spinal Cord Contusion // J. Neurosci. 2000. V. 20. № 17. P. 6421-6430.

[147] Huang D.W., McKerracher L., Braun P.E., David S. A therapeutic vaccine approach to stimulate axon regeneration in the adult mammalian spinal cord // Neuron. 1999. V. 24. № 3. P. 639-647.

[148] Kotter M.R., Li W.W., Zhao C., Franklin R.J. Myelin impairs CNS remyelination by inhibiting oligodendrocyte precursor cell differentiation // J. Neurosci. 2006. V. 26. № 1. P. 328-332.

[149] Taylor A.R., Welsh C.J., Young C., Spoor E., Kerwin S.C., Griffin J.F., Levine G.J., Cohen N.D., Levine J.M. Cerebrospinal fluid inflammatory cytokines and chemokines in naturally occurring canine spinal cord injury // J. Neurotrauma. 2014. V. 31. № 18. P. 1561-1569.

[150] Bradbury E.J., Burnside E.R. Moving beyond the glial scar for spinal cord repair // Nat. Commun. 2019. V. 10. P. 3879.

[151] Telegin G.B., Minakov A.N., Chernov A.S., Manskikh V.N.,

Asyutin D.S., Konovalov N.A., Gabibov A.G. Surgical Simulation of a Posttraumatic Spinal Cord Glial Scar in Rats // Acta Naturae. 2019. V. 11. № 3(42). P. 75-81.

[152] Sergeeva S.P., Erofeeva L.M., Gultyaev M.M., Balmasova I.P. Cytokines and cellular immune status after acute disorders of cerebral circulation // Immunopathology, Allergology, Infectology. 2010. № 3. P. 27-31.

[153] Belogurov A.A., Ivanova O.M., Lomakin Ya.A., Ziganshin R.Kh., Vaskina M.I., Knorre V.D., Klimova E.A., Gabibov A.G., Ivanov V .T., Govorun V.M. Mediators and biomarkers of inflammation in meningitis: cytokine and peptidome profiling of the cerebrospinal fluid // Biochemistry. 2016. Vol. 81. № 11. P. 1540-1552.

Chapter 2

Blood-Brain Barrier Dysfunction in the Detrimental Brain Function

Alejandro Gonzalez-Candia, Nicole K. Rogers and Rodrigo L. Castillo

Abstract

The blood circulation interface and the neural tissue feature unique characteristics encompassed by the term blood -brain barrier (BBB). The barrier's primary functions are maintenance of brain homeostasis, selective transport, and protection, all of them determined by its specialized multicellular structure. The BBB primarily exists at the level of the brain microvascular endothelium; however, endothelial cells are not intrinsically capable of forming a barrier. Indeed, the development of barrier characteristics in cerebral endothelial cells requires coordinated cell–cell interactions and signaling from glial cells (i.e., astrocytes, microglia), pericytes, neurons, and extracellular matrix. Such an intricate relationship implies the existence of a neurovascular unit (NVU). The NVU concept emphasizes that the dynamic BBB response to stressors requires coordinated interactions between various central nervous system (CNS) cell types and structures. Every cell type makes an indispensable contribution to the BBBs integrity, and any cell's failure or dysfunction might result in the barrier breakdown, with dramatic consequences, such as neuroinflammation and neurodegeneration. This chapter will focus on the structure and function of the BBB and discuss how BBB breakdown causes detrimental brain function.

Keywords: neurovascular unit, neurovascular coupling, BBB breakdown

1. Introduction

The interface between the blood circulation and the central nervous system (CNS) comprises complex multicellular structures with unique features that selectively allow or restrict the passage of substances between these compartments. Two distinct blood CNS barriers exist: the endothelial blood-brain barrier (BBB), localized at all levels of the cerebral vascular tree, and the epithelial blood-cerebrospinal fluid barrier, situated at the choroid plexuses within the brain's ventricular system, separating the brain interstitial fluid (ISF) and the cerebrospinal fluid (CSF) from the peripheral circulation [1].

The BBB is a term used to describe the unique properties of the microvasculature of CNS. The vascular tree are continuous non fenestrated vessels and contain a series of properties that allow them to tightly regulate the movement of molecules, ions, and cells between the blood and the CNS [2, 3]. The human brain is one of

IntechOpen

the most metabolically active organs in the body, under physiological conditions, the human brain receives 20% of the total basal cardiac output and uses 20% of the body's oxygen and glucose [4]. Energy substrates are consumed by the brain from the blood via transport across the BBB, as the brain lacks a metabolic reservoir to store macromolecules for use when needed. In the mammalian brain, cerebral arteries, arterioles, and capillaries supply CNS with blood in response to neuronal stimuli by increasing the rate of cerebral blood flow (CBF), nutrients and oxygen delivery, a mechanism known as neurovascular coupling [5].

The neurovascular coupling requires an integrated multicellular response to provide the perfusion needs for neuronal metabolism [5], different cell types are involved in this action, neurons and astrocytes generate mediators that trigger cellular responses in endothelium cells, pericytes, and smooth muscle cells (SMC), which contribute to vascular response in the BBB permeability. Functionally, these interactions are included in the concept of the neurovascular unit (NVU), which comprises various central and peripheral cell types that contribute to BBB structure and function (**Figure 1**) [6, 7]. However, in pathophysiological states, BBB breakdown and dysfunction leads to leakages of harmful blood components into the cerebral parenchyma, cellular infiltration, and aberrant transport and clearance of molecules [8], which is associated with CBF reductions and dysregulation [9], contributing to neurological effects.

Here, we first examine the cellular components that underlie the establishment of the BBB in NVU. Then, we focus on the cellular components of BBB and transport physiology. Complementary and in a translational way, examine how BBB breakdown and dysfunction related to acute vascular CNS disorders such as ischemic and hemorrhagic stroke, and BBB breakdown and dysfunction relate to neurological deficits and other pathologies in Alzheimer's disease (AD), Parkinson's disease (PD) and multiple sclerosis (MS).

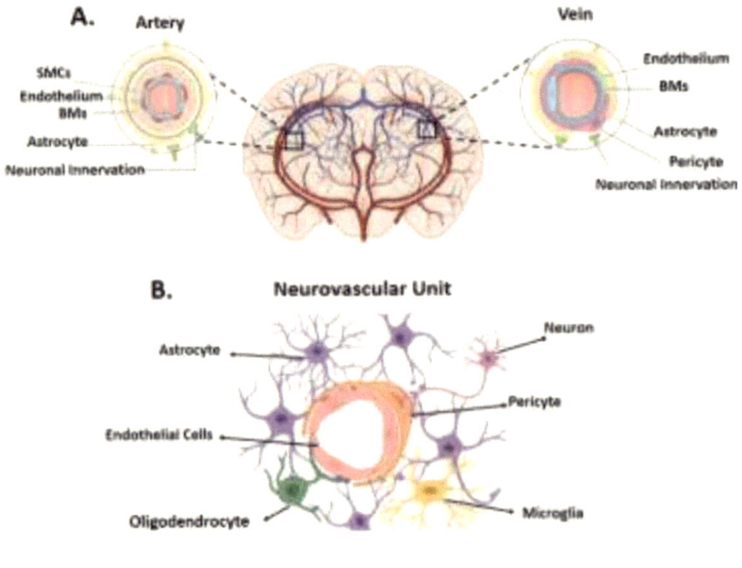

Figure 1.
(A) The multicellular structure of the neurovascular unit (NVU). The BBB is formed by endothelial cells at the level of the cerebral bed (arterial and venous). These endothelial cells interact with perivascular elements, such as the basal lamina (BMs), smooth muscle cells (SMCs) and astrocytic end-feet processes, perivascular neurons and pericytes to form a functional BBB. (B) The core anatomic elements of the NVU. Created with BioRender.com.

2. The BBB and the neurovascular unit

The NVU is a relatively recent neuroscience concept, representing the structural and functional multicellular relationship between the brain and blood vessels [5]. The cellular components are the endothelial cells (EC), pericytes, perivascular astrocytes, microglia, the basement membrane (BM), and neuron (**Figure 1**) [10]. The NVU components share intimate and complex associations, and these associations have led to their classification as a single functioning unit. The NVU is responsible for the maintenance of a highly selective BBB and cerebral homeostasis, as well as the control of CBF [11]. Each NVU component seems to play a specific and active role, maintaining the dynamic linkages reciprocally under physiological conditions.

Endothelial cells are considered the BBB's anatomic basis since they form and tightly seal the wall of all cerebral vessels, thereby building a physical barrier between the blood and the brain parenchyma (**Figure 1**). Two different types of endothelial junctions exist: adherens junctions (AJ) and tight junctions (TJ) [12]. Adherens junctions comprise vascular endothelial (VE) cadherin and neural (N-) cadherin, both acting via homophilic interactions [13]. While VE-cadherin is vital for sealing adjacent endothelial cells, N-cadherin mediates their association with pericytes [13]. TJ contains transmembrane proteins such as claudins, occludins, and junction adhesion molecules, as well as the zona occludens cytoplasmic proteins (ZO). These proteins act collectively to close off interconnecting endothelial cells [14], restricting the paracellular diffusion of hydrophilic substances, even ions; this is a unique feature of the BBB endothelium [11] in the other hand, the neurovascular endothelial cells, in contrast to peripheral endothelial cells, is the low expression of adhesion molecules (e.g. member of the immunoglobulin superfamily VCAM-1), in this sense, immune cells never cross unstimulated BBB in the healthy CNS [15]. Interactions of endothelial cells with other NVU members mediate a decrease in transcytotic activity, downregulation of leukocyte adhesion molecules, and regulation of interendothelial junction stability during development and adulthood [14].

Pericytes are mural cells enwrapping capillary blood vessels on their abluminal side. Structurally, pericytes extend processes from their cell body, covering several endothelial cells (**Figure 1**). In contrast to peripheral tissues, the brain has the highest pericyte to endothelial cell ratio [16]. Pericytes are embedded within the basement membrane (BM) of capillary endothelial cells and are thus centrally positioned between endothelial cells, astrocytes, and neurons [3]. In total, pericytes cover a large cerebral vascular area which can reach up to 40% of the neurovascular surface [17]. One of the main functions of pericytes is the control of the vasoreactivity and cerebral blood flow in response to neuronal activity [18]. As a recently explored example, glutamate induces prostaglandin E2 and nitric oxide release, which leads to actively relaxing pericytes to dilate capillaries [19]. Vascular permeability increases with decreasing pericyte coverage, which is partly due to the regulation of endothelial transcytosis. Moreover, other parts of the NVU are also influenced by pericytes, including neurons, immune cells, and the basement membrane [20].

Astrocytes are the most abundant cell type in the brain with a variety of functions. Beyond BBB regulation, they participate in synapse formation, uptake and recycling of neurotransmitters and ions, regulation of extracellular potassium levels, nutrition of neurons, and control of inflammatory responses within the CNS [21]. Astrocytes provide a cellular link between the neuronal circuitry and blood vessels. This neurovascular coupling enables astrocytes to relay signals that regulate blood flow in response to neuronal activity; this includes regulating the contraction/dilation of vascular SMC surrounding arterioles and capillaries [22, 23]. Astrocytes are also critical cellular support of BBB integrity. Recent molecular studies have shown several molecules released by astrocytes that enhance and maintain barrier tightness, such as cholesterol and phospholipid transporter molecule apolipoprotein E [24, 25]. Release of apolipoprotein E from astrocytes, for example, regulates endothelial TJs by signaling through the low-density lipoprotein receptor related protein 1 (LRP1) on both pericytes and endothelial cells of CNS microvessels [25]. Astrocytes have been identified as essential mediators of BBB formation and function because of purified astrocytes' ability to induce barrier properties in non-CNS blood vessels [26]. Based on these observations, it has been proposed that astrocytes are necessary for the formation of impermeable TJs in the developing vessels of the BBB.

Microglia derive from hematopoietic precursors that migrate from the yolk sac into the CNS parenchyma, acting as the brain's main line of defense past the BBB and play a vital role in innate immune responses in the vascular bed and cerebral parenchyma (**Figure 1**) [27], little is known about how microglial-endothelial communications may shape and regulate the homeostatic BBB. However, studies have demonstrated that microglia are associated with endothelial's nascent vessels in the developing brain, and promote the fusion of cells in the stages following vascular endothelial growth factor-mediated induction [28]. Recent studies have shown the activation of microglia in CNS disorders like AD and multiple sclerosis, which are associated with BBB breakdown and neuroinflammation. In these conditions, microglial activation may be both a cause and consequence of BBB dysfunction [20]. Microglia can exist in one of two active states: in the activated pathway, microglia release proinflammatory cytokines like interleukin-1b and tumor necrosis factor-a. Whereas in alternative pathways, microglia are involved in tissue repair, phagocytosing neurons and foreign material, releasing chemokines and vascular endothelial growth factor [29]. On the other hand, brain endothelial cells can also secrete molecules that cause microglial activation [30]. In summary, a complex interplay between systemic and CNS derived immune cells exists at the BBB.

Basement Membrane: The vascular tube is surrounded by two basement membranes (BMs), the inner vascular BM, and the outer parenchymal BM (**Figure 1**). The vascular BM is an extracellular matrix secreted by the ECs and pericytes, whereas the parenchymal BM is primarily secreted by astrocytic processes that extend towards the vasculature [31]. These BMs consist of different molecules, including type IV collagen, laminin, heparin sulfate proteoglycans, and other glycoproteins [32]. They provide an anchor for many signaling processes in the vasculature and also constitute an additional barrier for molecules and cells to cross before accessing the neural tissue. Disruption of these BMs by matrix metalloproteinases is an integral part of BBB dysfunction and posterior leukocyte infiltration, which can be observed in many different neurological disorders [32].

Neurons and interneurons. Neurons can detect small variations in their supply of nutrients and oxygen and transform these signals into electrical and chemical messages to adjacent interneurons or astrocytes. In response to these signals, necessary adjustment mechanisms are initiated. Due to this phenomenon, neurons are considered NVU's pacemaker [15]. Neurons need to be able to signal to cerebral vessels when their energy demands change. Positive and negative feedback mechanisms exist to regulate cerebral blood flow, accompanied by adjustments of substrate delivery across the BBB, a process known as neurovascular coupling [33]. In this sense, one relevant mechanism for neurovascular coupling is direct innervation of astrocytic processes or the endothelial tube by, amongst others, serotonergic, noradrenergic, cholinergic, and GABAergic neurons [4]. Mechanisms of neurovascular coupling, particularly those that can explain direct molecular effects on BBB integrity, are yet to be established. Future knowledge will be of great interest since new therapeutic tools could help modulate intercellular communication in diseases linked to vascular dysfunction.

3. BBB physiology: building blocks and transport routes in BBB

3.1 BBB junctional molecules

The BBB is a diffusion barrier essential for the normal function of the CNS. The NVU endothelial cells differ from endothelial cells in the rest of the vascular system by their absence of fenestrations, and for having more extensive junctional molecules, mainly TJ, and sparse pinocytic vesicular transport [34]. These junctional molecules limit the paracellular flux of hydrophilic molecules across the BBB. In contrast, small lipophilic substances (O2 or CO2) can diffuse freely across plasma membranes along their concentration gradient [34]. Nutrients such as glucose and amino acids enter the brain via transporters, whereas receptor-mediated endocytosis mediates larger molecules' uptake, including insulin, leptin, and iron transferrin [35], it is believed that all the components of the BBB are essential for the normal function, stability, and permeability of the BBB.

The Junction complex in the BBB comprises TJ, AJ, and Gap junctions (GJ). The TJ ultrastructurally appear as apparent fusion sites, involving the outer plasma membrane of adjacent endothelial cells [36]. The number of TJ strands, as well as the frequency of their ramifications, varies and consists of three integral membrane proteins: claudin, occludin, and junction adhesion molecules, as well as several other cytoplasmic accessory proteins, including members of the family zonula occludens (ZO-1, ZO-2, ZO-3) and cingulin (**Figure 2**). Cytoplasmic proteins link membrane proteins to actin, for maintaining the structural and functional integrity of the endothelium [36]. The Claudins were identified as the principal component of TJ and are localized exclusively at TJ strands. Claudins bind to other claudins on adjacent endothelial cells to form the primary seal of the TJ [37]. Closest to the

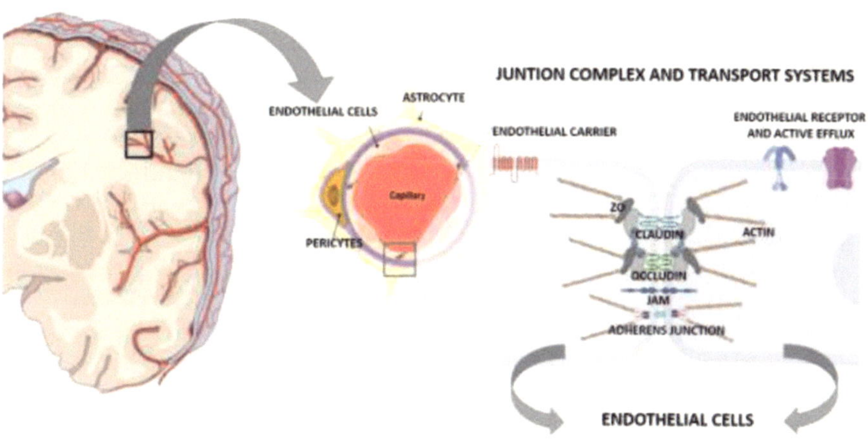

Figure 2.
Basic molecular organization of BBB junctional molecules and transport. The endothelial cells confer unique properties on the BBB. They are the principal line of cerebral vasculature and have numerous junctional molecules such as tight junctions, adherens junction, gap junctions and accessory proteins that limit the passive paracellular diffusion of all but the smallest of solutes and ions. On the other hand, carriers, receptors and active efflux protein mediated transport allow substances such as peptides, amino acids, and glucose to selectively cross the BBB and release toxic substances and drugs into the blood preventing them from entering the brain. Created with BioRender.com.

apical membrane, the claudin 1, 3, 5, 12, and occludins limit paracellular diffusion of solutes and ions across the BBB [38]. Loss of claudins is associated with permeability and BBB breakdown in neurodegenerative disorders and acute CNS diseases [39]. TJ proteins connect to actin and vinculin-based cytoskeletal filaments via scaffolding proteins of the membrane, associated with ZO 1, 2, and 3 [40]. Previous studies have shown that ZO-1 deficiency leads to BBB breakdown in many neurodegenerative and acute CNS disorders [41]. Occludin, another integral protein localized at the TJ, form the TJ's paracellular barrier when conjoined with neighboring cells' claudins [42]; the cytoplasmic domain of occludin directly associates with ZO proteins. The expression of occludin has also been documented in human adult brains, but not in average human newborn and fetal brain, suggesting their role as regulatory proteins that can alter paracellular permeability of the BBB [35]. The third type of TJ-associated membrane protein, junctional adhesion molecules (JAM), structurally consists of a single transmembrane domain and an extracellular portion with two immunoglobulin-like loops joined by disulfide bonds [43]. Three JAM-related proteins, JAM-1, JAM-2, and JAM-3 are expressed in human BBB and previous studies have shown their participation in cell-to-cell adhesion and monocyte transmigration through BBB [44].

The AJs are established between neighboring cells by homophilic interactions between the transmembrane proteins, vascular endothelial cadherin (VE-cadherin), and epithelial cadherin (E-cadherin) in CNS [13]. Nearby to the basolateral membrane, AJ proteins, VE-cadherin, and platelet endothelial cell adhesion molecule (PECAM-1) form homophilic endothelial-to-endothelial contacts limit paracellular diffusion of solutes [13]. GJ are other junctional molecules, whose connexin-37 (CX37), CX40, and CX43 form hemichannels between endothelial cells [45]. These membrane proteins enable direct cytoplasmic exchange of ions and low molecular weight metabolites between adjacent cells; these channels of communications are essential for propagating electrical signals and coordination of cell signaling by transfer of second messengers [46]. Furthermore, brain endothelial GP also support tight junction integrity.

3.2 BBB transport systems

The major BBB transporters, receptors, and channels found in endothelial cells and pericytes have been validated by transcriptomic studies and protein analysis (**Figure 2**) [34]. Except for gases and small lipophilic molecules that freely diffuse across the endothelium, brain endothelial transport systems regulate molecular exchanges between blood and brain. The BBB's highly selective nature and the high metabolic demand of the brain demand other routes of entry for various nutrients to feed and nurture the brain [34]. Metabolic supply is achieved via several transporters expressed on the surface of CNS endothelial cells that drive the active transport of specific solutes and metabolites into the brain [47]. On the other hand, given the close proximity and highly interactive signaling between vascular pericytes and endothelial cells, it is relevant to describe in this chapter the BBB pericyte transporter.

Endothelial carrier enables solutes such as carbohydrates, amino acids (AA), monocarboxylic acids, hormones, fatty acids, nucleotides, inorganic ions, amines, choline, and vitamins to cross the BBB via substrate-specific transporters (**Figure 2**). In terms of carbohydrate transporters, GLUT1 (glucose transporter 1) is a uniporter that transports glucose. GLUT1 can transport glucose (and other hexoses) from either side of the luminal and abluminal endothelial membrane extracellularly or intracellularly [48]. Since glucose is lower in the brain interstitial fluid (ISF) than plasma, GLUT1 favors blood-to-brain transport of circulating glucose. GLUT1 is expressed in endothelial cells, but not in neurons. Their importance is best illustrated by the fact that transcript encoding GLUT1 is one of the most abundant transcripts in brain endothelium. Their dysfunction and lack cause barrier breakdown and can prevent clearance of amyloid plaques, suggesting a contributing role in Alzheimer's disease progression [49].

Regarding the transport of amino acids, all essential AA are transported into the brain across the BBB via endothelial AA transporter 1 and 2 (LAT1/2), that transport bidirectionally neutral AA such as tryptophan and tyrosine [50], and the cationic AA transporter 1 and 3 (CAT1/3) that transport cationic AA such as lysine and arginine [51]. Also, on the abluminal membrane transporters for excitatory AA (EAAT1/2/3) transport glutamate and aspartate out of the brain, limiting their excitotoxic effects on neurons [52]. Transporters of neutral and excitatory AA, such as glycine, taurine, and GABA are enriched abluminally and with high-affinity transport from brain to endothelium in a sodium dependent manner, and then, these AA are transported across the luminal membrane of the BBB into the blood via low-affinity transporters into the circulation [53]. Finally, essential fatty acids are essential for brain development and postnatal neural functions. The Brain endothelium expresses luminal transporters for fatty acids, including fatty acid transport protein 1 and 4 (FATP- 1/4) and the MFSD2A (Major Facilitator Superfamily Domain containing 2a) [54]. In the brain, MFSD2a is exclusively expressed in brain endothelium and is required for right BBB development and functional integrity. Finally, for Lactate released from skeletal muscles during exercise, and ketone bodies derived from liver from metabolism of fatty acids, the transport is facilitated by monocarboxylate transporter-1 (MCT1). Once inside the brain parenchyma, they are used as alternative energy metabolites by the brain, supply the brain with key substrates for DNA and RNA synthesis [54]. Nucleotides and nitrogenous base, e.g., cytosine, guanine, adenine, thymine and uracil, are all transported across the BBB via sodium-independent concentrative nucleoside transporter-2 (CNT2) and the sodium-independent equilibrative nucleoside transporter-1 and 2 (ENT1/2) [55].

Endothelial receptor is the most important transporter because proteins and large macromolecules (e.g., fibrinogen, immunoglobulins, thrombin, plasminogen, and growth factors) cannot cross the BBB. However, some proteins and peptides use receptor transport to cross the BBB and enter the brain (**Figure 2**). Transferrin receptor (TfR) [56], insulin receptor (IR) [57], and leptin receptor (LEP-R) [58] mediate blood-to-brain transport of transferrin (iron-protein carrier), insulin, and leptin across the BBB, respectively. This characteristic has promoted its use for CNS drug delivery, including therapeutic antibodies [59]. Receptors LRP1 and LRP2 are expressed in the BBB's brain endothelium, with LRP1 binding Alzheimer's soluble Ab fragments and mediating its brain-to-blood clearance [60].

Endothelial active efflux and ion transport. ATP-binding cassette (ABC) transporters utilize ATP as an energy source and are expressed at the luminal side of the BBB endothelium. They function to prevent brain accumulation of drugs, xenobiotics and macromolecules via active efflux from endothelium to blood [**Figure 2**]. Some examples are ABCB1 (also known as P-glycoprotein, P-gp), breast cancer resistance protein (BCRP), and multidrug resistance-associated proteins (MRP). The BBB also has a significant role in regulating ions' concentration in the CNS. The luminal sodium pump, $Na^{+}K^{+}$ATPase, is a key regulator of sodium influx into the brain and potassium efflux from the brain, maintaining high concentrations of Na^{+} and low concentrations of K^{+} in the brain, critical for the electrophysiological equilibrium of the resting membrane and action potentials [61].

Luminal Na-K- Cl (chloride) cotransporter (NKCC) mediates entry of Na^{+}, K^{+} and $2Cl^{-}$ from blood-to-endothelium. The bicarbonate $(HCO_3)^{-}Cl$ exchanger mediates the entry of intracellular Cl^- and the extracellular release of HCO_3^-, regulating intracellular endothelial pH levels [62]. The Na^+-Ca^{2+} (sodium-calcium) exchanger cotransporter mediates Ca^{2+} efflux from endothelium into brain ISF, which maintains low intracellular Ca^{2+} levels in the microvascular endothelium [34]. Abluminal transient receptor potential (TRP) channels, also known as non- selective Ca^{2+} conducting cation channels, are expressed in both arterial endothelium and brain microvascular endothelial cell lines. TRP channels regulate Ca2 influx into brain endothelium, which in turn promotes the release of soluble factors such as NO, prostaglandins, and endothelial-derived hyperpolarizing factor initiating endothelium-dependent vasodilation [63]. BBB dysfunction also generates a leak of molecules across it, enabling considerable vascular fluid movement across the microvascular endothelium and the development of vasogenic edema [64]. Increased expression and activity of Na-K-Cl cotransporter (NKCC), sodium-hydrogen antiporter 1 and 2 (NHE1 and NHE2), and TRP channels promote the influx of Na^+, and Cl^-, generating a subsequent gradient osmotical that force the water movement across the BBB.

Pericyte transporters. Recent studies suggest that pericytes also express several transporters, receptors, and ion channels (**Figure 2**), such as carbohydrate transporters like the insulin-regulated glucose transporter GLUT4 and GLUT10 [65] and AA transporters, including the high-affinity excitatory AA transporter EAAT2, sodium-dependent neutral AA transporter SLC6A17, sodium and chloride dependent transporter SLC6A20 for small AA including glycine and proline, GABA transporter-1 and 2 (GAT1; GAT2), and the cationic AA transporter CAT2 [34, 65]. These transporters contribute to the removal of excitatory AA from the brain to prevent excitotoxicity, similar to endothelial transporters.

As endothelial cells, pericytes express lipoprotein receptor LRP1, mediating cellular uptake followed by its intracellular degradation and clearance [66] Pericytes regulate cerebrovascular integrity in an APOE-dependent way, inhibiting the proinflammatory CypA-MMP-9 pathway which prevents the degradation of BBB's TJ and basement membrane proteins [67]. These findings support that pericytes play an active role in regulating CBF and permeability of the BBB.

4. BBB dysfunction

BBB's integrity is essential for the normal functioning of the nervous system. It comes as no surprise then that its disruption initiates and perpetuates several neurological pathophysiological events. Although the nature and extent of such changes vary from every condition, one key commonality is the breakdown of BBB and the detrimental functioning of the NVU [4]. The BBB prevents neurotoxic plasma components, blood cells, and pathogens from entering the brain (integrity of BBB). At the same time, the BBB regulates transport of molecules into and out of the central nervous system (CNS) (permeability of BBB). In cerebrovascular diseases, BBB breakdown and dysfunction leads to leakages of components into the CNS, contributing to neurological deficits [68].

The cells of the NVU are extremely sensitive to a number of different substances, including pro-inflammatory cytokines (e.g. IL-1, IL-6, TNF-α, interferon-γ), lipid mediators, oxidative compounds (free radical), vasogenic agents (e.g. glutamate, serotonin, histamine) and other endogenous stimuli (e.g. extracellular K^+ and intracellular Ca^{2+}). Many of these substances are released under pathophysiological conditions and changes of their levels in BBB is a critical event in the development and progression of CNS dysfunction [69]. In some cases, increased BBB permeability is a consequence of the pathology, such as with ischemic stroke and traumatic brain injury, increased of intrinsic cellular proinflammatory, oxidative stress and dysregulation of vasogenic mediators, whereas in other cases BBB opening may be another condition in which cerebrovascular abnormalities have been noted, such as neurodegenerative disease [70]. As a result, there is a direct association between integrity impairment and high permeability of these substances in the brain. Some of the steps that follow include alteration or breakdown of the physical, transport, and immune barriers.

4.1 Alteration of BBB by cerebrovascular injury

4.1.1 Ischemic stroke

In ischemic stroke, there is a sudden cessation of blood supply to the brain tissue, which translates into reduced oxygen and glucose delivery, both essential for ATP production. Depletion of ATP levels can lead to impaired functioning of Na/K-ATPase and Ca^{+2}ATPase activity, generating ion- gradient failure and abnormal intracellular ion accumulation. By contrast, endothelial transporters' activity, such as Na/H ion-exchanger and Na-K-Cl cotransporter are stimulated. This secondarily induces increased Na^{+}, Cl^{-}, and water across to the barrier and into the brain parenchyma, which results in characteristic cytotoxic edema secondary to ischemia [71]. The stimulation of this transporter's activity also triggers endothelial cell Na^{+} accumulation, generating swelling that contributes to BBB breakdown [72]. The Na^{+} cellular uptake depolarizes the cell's membrane, opening voltage-gated ion channels and promoting Ca^{2+} further cell uptake. These changes, in turn, prompt the release of excitatory neurotransmitters, which can be toxic [71]. BBB's breakdown in stroke occurs in a biphasic subacute fashion [70]. In the initial hit, activated metalloproteinases MMP-2 attack tight junction proteins. This activation is mediated by membrane-type MMP (MMP-14) and the fur gene expression, regulated by hypoxia-induced factor 1a (HIF-1a) [73]. Decreased expression and disorganization of tight junction constituent proteins, claudins, are the first signs of BBB damage, with further dysfunction of influx and efflux BBB transporters' expression. These changes are limit the hypoxic area and revert after the acute insult [70].

After 24 and 48 hours post-reperfusion, a non-reversible second phase takes place. Proinflammatory local cytokines activate inducible and freely available metalloproteinases MMP-3 and MMP-9, whose destructive activity characterizes this phase [74]. The most abundant cytokines present in focal cerebral ischemic areas are TNF-alfa and IL-1b [75] and have also been observed to decrease the expression of occludin and ZO-1 [76]. Cyclooxygenase-2 also plays a role in this second and more harmful opening of the BBB. Although this inflammation is local and mainly initiated by the activation of glia and pericytes, the BBB's damage and opening allow monocytes and neutrophils' entrance, perpetuating and amplifying the local inflammatory response [74]. The breakage of BBB in ischemic stroke is also the precursor of further complications such as the hemorrhagic transformation of the infarcted parenchyma [77]. A schematic view of ischemic stroke and intracerebral hemorrhage mechanisms are shown in **Figure 3**.

BBB can also be disrupted by the action of reactive oxygen species (ROS) and ensuing oxidative stress. Superoxide anion (O^{2-}) is a known mediator of cellular damage after ischemic stroke. Under oxidative stress conditions such as stroke, superoxide dismutase's (SOD) metabolic capacity of controlling the biological activity of O^{2-} gets surpassed. When combined with nitric oxide (NO), O^{2-} forms peroxynitrite, a cytotoxic and proinflammatory molecule that can initiate and amplify BBB's injury by its ability to nitrosylate tyrosine and inducing endothelial damage [78]. Oxidative stress plays a critical role in ischemia/reperfusion (I/R)

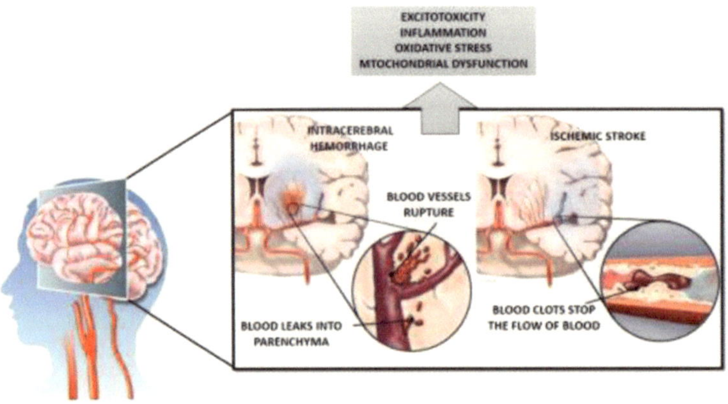

Figure 3.
A schematic view of ischemic stroke and intracerebral hemorrhage mechanisms. Activation of glutamate receptors following ischemic stroke leads to excitotoxicity and calcium influx, this impairs the neuronal homeostasis leading to activation of several calcium dependent pathways that include proteases and nucleases. Reperfusion aggravates the cerebral parenchyma damage by forming free radicals that damage the membranes and proteins. Further, the opening of mitochondrial permeability transition pore releases various proapoptotic molecules that activate apoptotic cell death in cerebral parenchyma. In intracerebral hemorrhage the initial bleed causes physical disruption of the cellular architecture of the brain and the mass of the haematoma may increase intracranial pressure which can compress brain regions, increasing neuronal death result of necrotic and apoptotic mechanisms depending on the severity of insult. Created with BioRender.com.

induced brain injury by stroke, various mechanisms in the neurovascular bed can trigger oxidative stress, including mitochondrial dysfunction, increase vasogenic mediators, glutamate release, and depletion of antioxidant defense system. Mitochondria are both important intracellular organelles for energy metabolism organelles, the main intracellular source of ROS, and important targets for I/R brain injury [79]. During stroke, inflammatory cytokines, oxidative stress, and Ca^{+2} overload stimulate the mitochondria, inducing the production of higher ROS levels, thereby triggering the mitochondrial necrosis pathway and leading to cell death [80]. In addition, endothelial cells, and immune cells produce large amounts of ROS during the cerebral ischemia phase, which in turn induce the activation of nuclear factor-κappa B (NF-κB), inducible endothelial nitric oxide (iNOS), and proinflammatory factors, triggering the upregulation of vascular endothelial cell adhesion molecules and causing BBB permeability [81].

4.1.2 Intracerebral hemorraghe

Between 10 and 15% of all strokes in the USA are intracerebral hemorrhages, which has higher morbidity and mortality when compared to ischemic strokes. Multiple etiologies are associated with ICH, hypertension being the more common, followed by amyloid pathology, especially in older populations, vascular malformations, and coagulopathies [72]. After the initial bleed, there can be a continuous bleed for the next 24 hours, the so-called hematoma expansion. A delayed vascular disruption occurs after the first 24 hours; this includes BBB dysfunction, which can associate with edema formation and an influx of leukocytes into the brain parenchyma [82].

The role of ischemia in ICH-induced brain injury is controversial, as a reduction in blood flow may be a result rather than the cause of brain damage. This suggests that BBB's increased permeability is due to the direct effect of certain blood components (thrombin, fibrin, and hemoglobin, iron) or to the inflammatory response to these components [72]. This phenomenon may include further peripheral cell infiltration and microglia activation, which may promote the higher secretion of proinflammatory cytokines and the activation of MMPs, as previously described in ischemic stroke [83].

4.2 Alteration of BBB by neurological disorders

4.2.1 Alzheimer's disease

Alzheimer's disease (AD) pathological hallmark is the accumulation of amyloid beta plaque deposits, which suggests the imbalance between its production and clearance rates may be due to a leaky BBB. The BBB dysfunction itself can also promote and accelerate the process of further AB production [84]. Diminished expression and dysfunction of ABC transporters at the BBB have been found in AD mice models [85], and two crucial BBB transporters in Abeta BBB's flow dynamics, p-glycoprotein LRP1, and RAGE have been identified as functionally impaired in AD. Expression of LRP1, which is in charge of the efflux of brain-derived Ab into blood across the BBB, is remarkably low at the BBB in AD patients' and AD models' brains [86]. Verapamil-PET studies in patients with mild AD, an exam that clinically assesses p-glycoprotein function, have found reduced activity of this transport in frontal, posterior cingulate, and the parietooccipital cortices, as well as in the hippocampus [87]. RAGE is a vital transporter that regulates the influx of circulating soluble ab intro the brain, which may promote neuroinflammation. Patients with AD develop increased levels of this transporter receptor both in brain endothelium and mural cells of the BBB [88].

There is enough evidence that associates AD with vascular disease at a pathological level [89]. Cerebral vessel pathology is not only a significant risk factor for AD but can also cause BBB disruption, as is the case with cerebral amyloid angiopathy [90]. Furthermore, changes in vascular biomarkers have been observed in preclinical AD before the development of cognitive impairment, and even before increases in routine AD biomarkers [91]. These findings support the two-hit vascular hypothesis of AD suggests that BBB dysfunction and brain hypoperfusion secondary to blood vessel damage may be the first hit that leads to ab accumulation and neuronal injury [92]. There is also evidence that at least two out of three BBB's main three cell lines are significantly compromised in AD. Accelerated pericyte degeneration and BBB breakdown is a distinguishing characteristic of AD-ApoE4 carriers mouse models [93]. On the other hand, astrocytic dysfunction, which has also been seen in AD models [84], may explain the hyperactivity of RAGE and hypoactivity of LRP1 in these patients' BBB. The pericyte degeneration initiates multiple pathways of neurodegeneration owing to the entry of several neurotoxic blood-derived proteins, including plasminogen, thrombin and fibrinogen which enter different areas of the CNS [93]. Plasmin, which is generated from circulating plasminogen, degrades the neuronal matrix protein laminin, thereby promoting neuronal injury. High concentrations of thrombin mediate neurotoxicity and memory impairment and accelerate BBB disruption [94].

4.2.2 Parkinson's disease

PD is one of the most prevalent neurodegenerative diseases after AD. It is characterized by filamentous and oligomeric α-synuclein (α-syn) accumulation, and degeneration of dopaminergic neurons in the substantia nigra leading to motor impairments [34]. Ever since the publication of Braak et al. studies, there is consensus that Parkinson's disease starts in the peripheral system and reaches the central nervous system in a retrograde (axon terminal to soma) spread of Lewy pathology.

Some authors have suggested that this spread could be through a hematogenous pathway [95]. Although PD patients in Braak stage 1 have their axon terminals outside the BBB, this same structure protects the somas of those axons, which reside in the central nervous system. Cerebrovascular disease also plays a part in PD, as both vascular disease and vascular risk factors aggravate motor and cognitive symptoms [96]. This may explain the BBB leakiness observed in these patients, as a recent study observed in the post-commissural putamen of PD patients, using histologic markers of serum protein, iron, and erythrocyte extravasation [97]. Regarding the extravasation of molecules through the cerebral vascular system, the histological analysis of PD patients reveals BBB breakdown in the striatum as shown by capillary leakages and accumulation of perivascular fibrinogen, immunoglobulins deposits, hemosiderin, red blood cells extravasation and leukocyte infiltration [98]. Increased BBB permeability and inducing inflammatory and necrotic processes in the brain parenchyma.

In patients with PD, a dysregulation of the transport systems has also been observed in the BBB, recent studies reveal that α-syn crosses the BBB, which could signify an important contributory event in PD pathogenesis (neurodegeneration) [99]. The α-syn oligomers crossed the BBB into the brain, in parenchyma where α-syn amplification and strain-specific pathology and neurotoxic phenotypes. In the other hand, regarding the clearance of the α-syn, this molecule is capable of inhibiting Aβ efflux suggesting and the endothelial LRP1 is a only potential efflux transporter for α-syn, however, LRP1 is similarly downregulated in PD [100], this could result in impaired α-syn BBB clearance and accumulation in brain, suggesting that the high levels of α-syn produced peripherally can enter the brain in the presence of BBB breakdown, which may also contribute to development of PD pathology.

4.2.3 Multiple sclerosis

Multiple sclerosis (MS) is an autoimmune disease with an early BBB disruption pattern. One clear indication is the presence of Gadolinium-enhancing lesions on magnetic resonance, which translates in extravasation of intravascular contrast due to brain parenchyma and its associated active inflammation. Moreover, an increasing amount of evidence shows this disruption could not be restricted to Gd-enhancing lesions, as observed in non-enhancing areas in postmortem MS brains [101]. As the entry of inflammatory infiltrate occurs in the brain's perivascular regions, it is intuitive to think BBB disruption is very likely an early event in lesion formation.

There is also evidence of maladaptive changes in the NVU's components. One great example is ECs, which upregulate adhesion molecules and display chemokines on their luminal surface, to promote transcellular immune cell migration [102]. Also, in MS, TJ abnormalities can be seen, as one study observed abnormal ZO-1 at TJs in sections of primary progressive MS patients' cortical grey matter [101]. The BM in these patients' lesions also appears discontinuous. MRI studies have shown hypoperfusion in early and advanced stages of MS, suggesting the presence of metabolic injury in the brain parenchyma in a hypoxia-like fashion [103]. Regarding a primary BBB dysfunction, studies have focused on astrocytes and pericytes, whose maladaptive changes could explain the reduction in capillary blood flow and further hypoxia. D'haeseleer et al. observed that the hypoperfusion in MS could be mediated by astrocyte's released endothelin-1 (ET-1), as it can be normalized with an ET-1 antagonist [104]. This body of evidence conveys heterogeneous pathophysiology in MS, one that included BBB breakdown as a primary event and not only as a secondary consequence [105].

5. Conclusion and future directions

The relevance of the NVU in the support of cerebral homeostasis of the BBB is being partly established with recent evidence. The multifactorial interactions between their components are extremely refined, expressing the complexity of the central CNS physiology. The knowledge of each of the components and their respective pathways are critical to understanding various neurovascular diseases, such as cerebrovascular injury (e.g. stroke) and neurological disorders (e.g. Alzheimer's). Although despite current knowledge, many questions about the role of each component NVU, pathways and crosstalking still have no answer. These advances have uncovered gaps in our knowledge of neurovascular health and have provided us with the roadmap to ask new questions that should be addressed by the future studies. Finally, based on the current state of our knowledge, it is probably time to think about BBB not only as an impermeable cellular membrane which protects brain from peripheral influences and should be breached for therapeutic CNS drug delivery, but also as an enormous source of understudied molecular and cellular targets in the pathophysiological states, which if explored could change the paradigm about brain diseases therapy and could lead to development of novel BBB-based personalized approaches to treat them.

Author details

Alejandro Gonzalez-Candia[1], Nicole K. Rogers[2] and Rodrigo L. Castillo[3,4]*

1 Institute of Health Sciences, University of O'Higgins, Rancagua, Chile

2 Department of Neuroscience, Faculty of Medicine, University of Chile, Santiago, Chile

3 Department of Internal Medicine East Division, Faculty of Medicine, University of Chile, Santiago, Chile

4 Critical Patient Unit, Hospital del Salvador, Santiago, Chile

*Address all correspondence to: rodrigouch@uchile.cl; rodrigouch@gmail.com

References

[1] Tumani H, Huss A, Bachhuber F. The cerebrospinal fluid and barriers anatomic and physiologic considerations. Handbook of Clinical Neurology. 2017;**146**:21-32. DOI: 10.1016/B978-0-12-804279-3.00002-2

[2] Pandit R, Chen L, Götz J. The blood-brain barrier: Physiology and strategies for drug delivery [published online ahead of print, 2019 Nov 29]. Adv Drug Deliv Rev. 2019; S0169-409X (19)30238-8. doi: 10.1016/j.addr.2019.11.009.

[3] Liebner S, Dijkhuizen RM, Reiss Y, Plate KH, Agalliu D, Constantin G. Functional morphology of the blood-brain barrier in health and disease. Acta Neuropathologica. 2018;**135**(3):311-336. DOI: 10.1007/s00401-018-1815-1

[4] Obermeier B, Daneman R, Ransohoff RM. Development, maintenance and disruption of the blood-brain barrier. Nature Medicine. 2013;**19**(12):1584-1596. DOI: 10.1038/nm.3407

[5] Iadecola C. The Neurovascular Unit Coming of Age: A Journey through Neurovascular Coupling in Health and Disease. Neuron. 2017;**96**(1):17-42. DOI: 10.1016/j.neuron.2017.07.030

[6] Phillips AA, Chan FH, Zheng MM, Krassioukov AV, Ainslie PN. Neurovascular coupling in humans: Physiology, methodological advances and clinical implications. Journal of Cerebral Blood Flow and Metabolism. 2016;**36**(4):647-664. DOI: 10.1177/0271678X15617954

[7] Filosa JA, Morrison HW, Iddings JA, Du W, Kim KJ. Beyond neurovascular coupling, role of astrocytes in the regulation of vascular tone. Neuroscience. 2016;**323**:96-109. DOI: 10.1016/j.neuroscience.2015.03.064

[8] Engelhardt B, Sorokin L. The blood-brain and the blood-cerebrospinal fluid barriers: function and dysfunction. Seminars in Immunopathology. 2009;**31**(4):497-511. DOI: 10.1007/s00281-009-0177-0

[9] Goldwaser EL, Acharya NK, Sarkar A, Godsey G, Nagele RG. Breakdown of the Cerebrovasculature and Blood-Brain Barrier: A Mechanistic Link Between Diabetes Mellitus and Alzheimer's Disease. Journal of Alzheimer's Disease. 2016;**54**(2):445-456. DOI: 10.3233/JAD-160284

[10] Langen UH, Ayloo S, Gu C. Development and Cell Biology of the Blood-Brain Barrier. Annual Review of Cell and Developmental Biology. 2019;**35**:591-613. DOI: 10.1146/annurev-cellbio-100617-062608

[11] Muoio V, Persson PB, Sendeski MM. The neurovascular unit concept review. Acta Physiologica (Oxford, England). 2014;**210**(4):790-798. DOI: 10.1111/apha.12250

[12] Dejana E, Giampietro C. Vascular endothelial-cadherin and vascular stability. Current Opinion in Hematology. 2012;**19**(3):218-223. DOI: 10.1097/MOH.0b013e3283523e1c

[13] Tietz S, Engelhardt B. Brain barriers: Crosstalk between complex tight junctions and adherens junctions. The Journal of Cell Biology. 2015;**209**(4):493-506. DOI: 10.1083/jcb.201412147

[14] Blanchette M, Daneman R. Formation and maintenance of the BBB. Mechanisms of Development. 2015;**138**(Pt 1):8-16. DOI: 10.1016/j.mod.2015.07.007

[15] Obermeier B, Verma A, Ransohoff RM. The blood-brain barrier. Handbook of Clinical Neurology.

2016;**133**:39-59. DOI: 10.1016/B978-0-444-63432-0.00003-7

[16] Brown LS, Foster CG, Courtney JM, King NE, Howells DW, Sutherland BA. Pericytes and Neurovascular Function in the Healthy and Diseased Brain. Front Cell Neurosci. 2019; 13:282. Published 2019 Jun 28. doi:10.3389/fncel.2019.00282.

[17] Mathiisen TM, Lehre KP, Danbolt NC, Ottersen OP. The perivascular astroglial sheath provides a complete covering of the brain microvessels: an electron microscopic 3D reconstruction. Glia. 2010;**58**(9):1094-1103. DOI: 10.1002/glia.20990

[18] Peppiatt CM, Howarth C, Mobbs P, Attwell D. Bidirectional control of CNS capillary diameter by pericytes. Nature. 2006;**443**(7112):700-704. DOI: 10.1038/nature05193

[19] Hill J, Rom S, Ramirez SH, Persidsky Y. Emerging roles of pericytes in the regulation of the neurovascular unit in health and disease. Journal of Neuroimmune Pharmacology. 2014;**9**(5):591-605. DOI: 10.1007/s11481-014-9557-x

[20] Keaney J, Campbell M. The dynamic blood-brain barrier. The FEBS Journal. 2015;**282**(21):4067-4079. DOI: 10.1111/febs.13412

[21] Armulik A, Genové G, Mäe M, et al. Pericytes regulate the blood-brain barrier. Nature. 2010;**468**(7323):557-561. DOI: 10.1038/nature09522

[22] Nuriya M, Hirase H. Involvement of astrocytes in neurovascular communication. Progress in Brain Research. 2016;**225**:41-62. DOI: 10.1016/bs.pbr.2016.02.001

[23] Tait MJ, Saadoun S, Bell BA, Papadopoulos MC. Water movements in the brain: role of aquaporins. Trends in Neurosciences. 2008;**31**:37-43. DOI: 10.1016/j.tins.2007.11.003

[24] WosikK,CayrolR,Dodelet-DevillersA, Berthelet F, Bernard M, Moumdjian R, et al. Angiotensin II controls occludin function and is required for blood-brain barrier maintenance: relevance to multiple sclerosis. The Journal of Neuroscience. 2007;**27**:9032-9042. DOI: 10.1523/JNEUROSCI.2088-07.2007

[25] Bell RD, Winkler EA, Singh I, Sagare AP, Deane R, Wu Z, et al. Apolipoprotein E controls cerebrovascular integrity via cyclophilin A. Nature. 2012;**485**:512-551. DOI: 10.1038/nature11087

[26] Daneman R, Prat A. The blood-brain barrier. Cold Spring Harb Perspect Biol. 2015;7(1): a020412. Published 2015 Jan 5. doi:10.1101/cshperspect.a020412.

[27] Ginhoux F, Greter M, Leboeuf M, Nandi S, See P, Gokhan S, et al. Fate mapping analysis reveals that adult microglia derive from primitive macrophages. Science. 2010;**330**:841-845. DOI: 10.1126/science.1194637

[28] Fantin A, Vieira JM, Gestri G, Denti L, Schwarz Q, Prykhozhij S, et al. Tissue macrophages act as cellular chaperones for vascular anastomosis downstream of VEGF-mediated endothelial tip cell induction. Blood. 2010;**116**:829-840. DOI: 10.1182/blood-2009-12-257832

[29] Ju F, Ran Y, Zhu L, Cheng X, Gao H, Xi X, et al. Increased BBB Permeability Enhances Activation of Microglia and Exacerbates Loss of Dendritic Spines After Transient Global Cerebral Ischemia. Frontiers in Cellular Neuroscience. 2018;**12**:236. DOI: 10.3389/fncel.2018.00236

[30] Yin X, Wright J, Wall T, Grammas P. Brain endothelial cells synthesize neurotoxic thrombin in Alzheimer's disease. The American

Journal of Pathology. 2010;**176**:1600-1606. DOI: 10.2353/ajpath.2010.090406

[31] Thomsen MS, Routhe LJ, Moos T. The vascular basement membrane in the healthy and pathological brain. Journal of Cerebral Blood Flow and Metabolism. 2017;**37**(10):3300-3317. DOI: 10.1177/0271678X17722436

[32] Xu L, Nirwane A, Yao Y. Basement membrane and blood-brain barrier. Stroke Vasc Neurol. 2018;**4**(2):78-82. DOI: 10.1136/svn-2018-000198

[33] Leybaert L. Neurobarrier coupling in the brain: a partner of neurovascular and neurometabolic coupling? Journal of Cerebral Blood Flow and Metabolism. 2005;**25**(1):2-16. DOI: 10.1038/sj.jcbfm.9600001

[34] Sweeney MD, Zhao Z, Montagne A, Nelson AR, Zlokovic BV. Blood-Brain Barrier: From Physiology to Disease and Back. Physiological Reviews. 2019;**99**(1):21-78. DOI: 10.1152/physrev.00050.2017

[35] Ballabh P, Braun A, Nedergaard M. The blood-brain barrier: an overview: structure, regulation, and clinical implications. Neurobiology of Disease. 2004;**16**(1):1-13. DOI: 10.1016/j.nbd.2003.12.016

[36] Greene C, Campbell M. Tight junction modulation of the blood brain barrier: CNS delivery of small molecules. Tissue Barriers. 2016;**4**(1):e1138017. DOI: 10.1080/21688370.2015.1138017

[37] Furuse M, Fujita K, Hiiragi T, Fujimoto K, Tsukita S. Claudin-1 and -2: novel integral membrane proteins localizing at tight junctions with no sequence similarity to occludin. The Journal of Cell Biology. 1998;**141**:1539-1550. DOI: 10.1083/jcb.141.7.1539

[38] Nitta T, Hata M, Gotoh S, Seo Y, Sasaki H, Hashimoto N, et al. Size-selective loosening of the blood-brain barrier in claudin-5-deficient mice. The Journal of Cell Biology. 2003;**161**:653-660. DOI: 10.1083/jcb.200302070

[39] Zlokovic BV. The blood-brain barrier in health and chronic neurodegenerative disorders. Neuron. 2008;**57**:178-201. DOI: 10.1016/j.neuron.2008.01.003

[40] Van Itallie CM, Anderson JM. Architecture of tight junctions and principles of molecular composition. Seminars in Cell & Developmental Biology. 2014;**36**:157-165. DOI: 10.1016/j.semcdb.2014. 08.011

[41] Zlokovic BV. Neurovascular pathways to neurodegeneration in Alzheimer's disease and other disorders. Nature Reviews. Neuroscience. 2011;**12**:723-738. DOI: 10.1038/nrn3114

[42] Reinhold AK, Rittner HL. Barrier function in the peripheral and central nervous system-a review. Pflügers Archiv. 2017;**469**(1):123-134. DOI: 10.1007/s00424-016-1920-8

[43] Dejana E, Lampugnani MG, Martinez-Estrada O, Bazzoni G. The molecular organization of endothelial junctions and their functional role in vascular morphogenesis and permeability. The International Journal of Developmental Biology. 2000;**44**:743-748

[44] Hawkins BT, Davis TP. The blood-brain barrier/neurovascular unit in health and disease. Pharmacological Reviews. 2005;**57**(2):173-185. DOI: 10.1124/pr.57.2.4

[45] Nagasawa K, Chiba H, Fujita H, Kojima T, Saito T, Endo T, et al. Possible involvement of gap junctions in the barrier function of tight junctions of brain and lung endothelial cells. Journal of Cellular Physiology. 2006;**208**:123-132. DOI: 10.1002/jcp.20647

[46] Nielsen MS, Axelsen LN, Sorgen PL, Verma V, Delmar M, Holstein-Rathlou NH. Gap junctions. Comprehensive Physiology. 2012;**2**(3):1981-2035. DOI: 10.1002/cphy.c110051

[47] Erdő F, Krajcsi P. Age-Related Functional and Expressional Changes in Efflux Pathways at the Blood-Brain Barrier. Frontiers in Aging Neuroscience. 2019;**11**:196. DOI: 10.3389/fnagi.2019.00196

[48] Jurcovicova J. Glucose transport in brain effect of inflammation. Endocrine Regulations. 2014;**48**(1):35-48. DOI: 10.4149/endo_2014_01_35

[49] Winkler EA, Nishida Y, Sagare AP, Rege SV, Bell RD, Perlmutter D, et al. GLUT1 reductions exacerbate Alzheimer's disease vasculo-neuronal dysfunction and degeneration. Nature Neuroscience. 2015;**18**:521-530. DOI: 10.1038/nn.3966

[50] O'Kane RL, Hawkins RA. Na+ dependent transport of large neutral amino acids occurs at the abluminal membrane of the blood-brain barrier. American Journal of Physiology. Endocrinology and Metabolism. 2003;**285**:E1167-E1173. DOI: 10.1152/ajpendo.00193.2003

[51] Mann GE, Yudilevich DL, Sobrevia L. Regulation of amino acid and glucose transporters in endothelial and smooth muscle cells. Physiol Rev. 2003; 83: 183-252. doi:10. 1152/physrev.00022.2002.

[52] O'Kane RL, Martínez-López I, De Joseph MR, Viña JR, Hawkins RA. Na (+)-dependent glutamate transporters (EAAT1, EAAT2, and EAAT3) of the blood-brain barrier. A mechanism for glutamate removal. The Journal of Biological Chemistry. 1999;**274**:31891-31895. DOI: 10.1074/ jbc.274.45.31891

[53] Lee WJ, Hawkins RA, Viña JR, Peterson DR. Glutamine transport by the blood-brain barrier: a possible mechanism for nitrogen removal. American Journal of Physiology. Cell Physiology. 1998;**274**:C1101-C1107. DOI: 10.1152/ajpcell.1998.274.4.C1101

[54] Simpson IA, Carruthers A, Vannucci SJ. Supply and demand in cerebral energy metabolism: the role of nutrient transporters. Journal of Cerebral Blood Flow and Metabolism. 2007;**27**:1766-1791. DOI: 10.1038/sj.jcbfm.9600521

[55] Cass CE, Young JD, Baldwin SA. Recent advances in the molecular biology of nucleoside transporters of mammalian cells. Biochem Cell Biol. 1998; 76: 761-770. doi:10. 1139/o98-095.

[56] Jefferies WA, Brandon MR, Hunt SV, Williams AF, Gatter KC, Mason DY. Transferrin receptor on endothelium of brain capillaries. Nature. 1984; 312: 162-163. doi:10. 1038/312162a0.

[57] to S, Yanai M, Yamaguchi S, Couraud PO, Ohtsuki S. Regulation of Tight-Junction Integrity by Insulin in an in Vitro Model of Human Blood-Brain Barrier. J Pharm Sci. 2017; 106: 2599-2605. doi: 10.1016/j.xphs.2017.04.036.

[58] Golden PL, Maccagnan TJ, Pardridge WM. Human blood-brain barrier leptin receptor. Binding and endocytosis in isolated human brain microvessels. The Journal of Clinical Investigation. 1997;**99**:14-18. DOI: 10.1172/JCI119125

[59] Pardridge WM. Drug transport across the blood-brain barrier. Journal of Cerebral Blood Flow and Metabolism. 2012;**32**:1959-1972. DOI: 10.1038/jcbfm.2012.126

[60] Deane R, Singh I, Sagare AP, Bell RD, Ross NT, La Rue B, et al. A multimodal RAGE-specific inhibitor reduces amyloid-mediated brain disorder in a mouse model of Alzheimer disease. The Journal of Clinical

Investigation. 2012;**122**:1377-1392. DOI: 10.1172/ JCI58642

[61] Funck VR, Ribeiro LR, Pereira LM, de Oliveira CV, Grigoletto J, Della-Pace ID, et al. Contrasting effects of Na, K - ATPase activation on seizure activity in acute versus chronic models. Neuroscience. 2015;**298**:171-179. DOI: 10.1016/j.neuroscience.2015.04.031

[62] Taylor CJ, Nicola PA, Wang S, Barrand MA, Hladky SB. Transporters involved in regulation of intracellular pH in primary cultured rat brain endothelial cells. The Journal of Physiology. 2006;**576**:769-785. DOI: 10.1113/jphysiol.2006.117374

[63] Sonkusare SK, Bonev AD, Ledoux J, Liedtke W, Kotlikoff MI, Heppner TJ, Hill-Eu- banks DC, Nelson MT. Elementary Ca2 signals through endothelial TRPV4 channels regulate vascular function. Science 2012; 336: 597-601. doi:10.1126/science. 1216283.

[64] Jia SW, Liu XY, Wang SC, Wang YF. Vasopressin Hypersecretion-Associated Brain Edema Formation in Ischemic Stroke: Underlying Mechanisms. Journal of Stroke and Cerebrovascular Diseases. 2016;**25**(6):1289-1300. DOI: 10.1016/j. jstrokecerebrovasdis.2016.02.002

[65] Armulik A, Genové G, Mäe M, Nisancioglu MH, Wallgard E, Niaudet C, et al. Pericytes regulate the blood-brain barrier. Nature. 2010;**468**:557-561. DOI: 10.1038/nature09522

[66] Sagare AP, Bell RD, Zhao Z, Ma Q, Winkler EA, Ramanathan A, et al. Pericyte loss influences Alzheimer-like neurodegeneration in mice. Nature Communications. 2013;**4**:2932. DOI: 10.1038/ncomms3932

[67] Bell RD, Winkler EA, Singh I, Sagare AP, Deane R, Wu Z, et al. Apolipoprotein E controls cerebrovascular integrity via cyclophilin A. Nature. 2012;**485**:512-516. DOI: 10.1038/nature11087

[68] Schenk GJ, de Vries HE. Altered blood-brain barrier transport in neuro-inflammatory disorders. Drug Discovery Today: Technologies. 2016;**20**:5-11. DOI: 10.1016/j.ddtec.2016.07.002

[69] Worzfeld T, Schwaninger M. Apicobasal polarity of brain endothelial cells. Journal of Cerebral Blood Flow and Metabolism. 2016 Feb;**36**(2):340-362. DOI: 10.1016/j.ddtec.2016.07.002

[70] Rosenberg GA. Neurological diseases in relation to the blood-brain barrier. Journal of Cerebral Blood Flow and Metabolism. 2012;**32**(7):1139-1151. DOI: 10.1038/jcbfm.2011.197

[71] O'Donnell ME. Blood-brain barrier Na transporters in ischemic stroke. Advances in Pharmacology. 2014;**71**:113-146. DOI: 10.1016/ bs.apha.2014.06.011

[72] Keep RF, Andjelkovic AV, Stamatovic SM, Shakui P, Ennis SR. Ischemia-induced endothelial cell dysfunction. Acta Neurochirurgica. Supplement. 2005;**95**:399-402. DOI: 10.1007/3-211-32318-x_81

[73] Yang Y, Estrada EY, Thompson JF, Liu W, Rosenberg GA. Matrix metalloproteinase-mediated disruption of tight junction proteins in cerebral vessels is reversed by synthetic matrix metalloproteinase inhibitor in focal ischemia in rat. Journal of Cerebral Blood Flow and Metabolism. 2007;**27**(4):697-709. DOI: 10.1038/ sj.jcbfm.9600375

[74] Abdullahi W, Tripathi D, Ronaldson PT. Blood-brain barrier dysfunction in ischemic stroke: targeting tight junctions and transporters for vascular protection. American Journal of Physiology. Cell Physiology. 2018;**315**(3):C343-C356. DOI: 10.1152/ajpcell.00095.2018

[75] Boutin H, LeFeuvre RA, Horai R, Asano M, Iwakura Y, Rothwell NJ. Role of IL-1alpha and IL-1beta in ischemic brain damage [published correction appears in J Neurosci 2001 Sep 1;21(17):1a]. The Journal of Neuroscience. 2001;**21**(15):5528-5534. DOI: 10.1523/JNEUROSCI.21-15-05528.2001

[76] Rochfort KD, Cummins PM. Cytokine-mediated dysregulation of zonula occludens-1 properties in human brain microvascular endothelium. Microvascular Research. 2015;**100**:48-53. DOI: 10.1016/j.mvr.2015.04.010

[77] Kassner A, Merali Z. Assessment of Blood-Brain Barrier Disruption in Stroke. Stroke. 2015;**46**(11):3310-3315. DOI: 10.1161/STROKEAHA.115.008861

[78] Carvalho AN, Firuzi O, Gama MJ, Horssen JV, Saso L. Oxidative Stress and Antioxidants in Neurological Diseases: Is There Still Hope? Current Drug Targets. 2017;**18**(6):705-718. DOI: 10.2174/1389450117666160401120514

[79] Zhao XY, Lu MH, Yuan DJ, Xu DE, Yao PP, Ji WL, et al. Mitochondrial Dysfunction in Neural Injury. Frontiers in Neuroscience. 2019;**4**:13-30. DOI: 10.3389/fnins.2019.00030

[80] Zhu Y, Wang H, Fang J, Dai W, Zhou J, Wang X, et al. SS-31 Provides Neuroprotection by Reversing Mitochondrial Dysfunction after Traumatic Brain Injury. Oxidative Medicine and Cellular Longevity. 2018;**27**:4783602. DOI: 10.1155/2018/4783602

[81] Abdul-Muneer PM, Chandra N, Haorah J. Interactions of oxidative stress and neurovascular inflammation in the pathogenesis of traumatic brain injury. Molecular Neurobiology. 2015;**51**(3):966-979. DOI: 10.1007/s12035-014-8752-3

[82] Murai Y, Ikeda Y, Teramoto A, Tsuji Y. Magnetic resonance imaging-documented extravasation as an indicator of acute hypertensive intracerebral hemorrhage. Journal of Neurosurgery. 1998;**88**(4):650-655. DOI: 10.3171/jns.1998.88.4.0650

[83] Moxon-Emre I, Schlichter LC. Neutrophil depletion reduces blood-brain barrier breakdown, axon injury, and inflammation after intracerebral hemorrhage. Journal of Neuropathology and Experimental Neurology. 2011;**70**(3):218-235. DOI: 10.1097/NEN.0b013e31820d94a5

[84] Cai Z, Qiao PF, Wan CQ, Cai M, Zhou NK, Li Q. Role of Blood-Brain Barrier in Alzheimer's Disease. Journal of Alzheimer's Disease. 2018;**63**(4):1223-1234. DOI: 10.3233/JAD-180098

[85] Cirrito JR, Deane R, Fagan AM, Spinner ML, Parsadanian M, Finn MB, et al. P-glycoprotein deficiency at the blood-brain barrier increases amyloid-beta deposition in an Alzheimer disease mouse model. The Journal of Clinical Investigation. 2005;**115**:3285-3290. DOI: 10.1172/ JCI25247

[86] Deane R, Bell RD, Sagare A, Zlokovic BV. Clearance of amyloid-beta peptide across the blood-brain barrier: implication for therapies in Alzheimer's disease. CNS & Neurological Disorders Drug Targets. 2009;**8**(1):16-30. DOI: 10.2174/187152709787601867

[87] Deo AK, Borson S, Link JM, et al. Activity of P-Glycoprotein, a β-Amyloid Transporter at the Blood-Brain Barrier, Is Compromised in Patients with Mild Alzheimer Disease. Journal of Nuclear Medicine. 2014;**55**(7):1106-1111. DOI: 10.2967/jnumed.113.130161

[88] Donahue JE et al. RAGE, LRP-1, and amyloid-beta protein in Alzheimer's disease. Acta Neuropathol (Berl). 2006;**112**:405-415. DOI: 10.1007/s00401-006-0115-3

[89] Snowdon DA, Greiner LH, Mortimer JA, Riley KP, Greiner PA, Markesbery WR. Brain Infarction and the Clinical Expression of Alzheimer Disease: The Nun Study. Journal of the American Medical Association. 1997;**277**(10):813-817. DOI: 10.1001/jama.1997.03540340047031

[90] Saito S, Ihara M. Interaction between cerebrovascular disease and Alzheimer pathology. Current Opinion in Psychiatry. 2016;**29**(2):168-173. DOI: 10.1097/YCO.0000000000000239

[91] Iturria-Medina Y, Sotero RC, Toussaint PJ, Mateos-Pérez JM, Evans AC; Alzheimer's Disease Neuroimaging Initiative. Early role of vascular dysregulation on late-onset Alzheimer's disease based on multifactorial data-driven analysis. Nat Commun. 2016; 7:11934. doi: 10.1038/ncomms11934.

[92] Nelson AR, Sweeney MD, Sagare AP, Zlokovic BV. Neurovascular dysfunction and neurodegeneration in dementia and Alzheimer's disease. Biochimica et Biophysica Acta. 2016;**1862**(5):887-900. DOI: 10.1016/j.bbadis.2015.12.016

[93] Halliday MR, Rege SV, Ma Q, Zhao Z, Miller CA, Winkler EA, et al. Accelerated pericyte degeneration and blood-brain barrier breakdown in apolipoprotein E4 carriers with Alzheimer's disease. Journal of Cerebral Blood Flow and Metabolism. 2016;**36**:216-227. DOI: 10.1038/jcbfm.2015.44

[94] Sweeney M, Sagare A, Zlokovic B. Blood–brain barrier breakdown in Alzheimer disease and other neurodegenerative disorders. Nat Rev Neurol. 2018; 14: 133-150. doi.org/10.1038/nrneurol.2017.188.

[95] Woulfe JM, Gray MT, Gray DA, Munoz DG, Middeldorp JM. Hypothesis: a role for EBV-induced molecular mimicry in Parkinson's disease. Parkinsonism & Related Disorders. 2014;**20**:685-694. DOI: 10.1016/j.parkreldis.2014.02.031

[96] Malek N, Lawton MA, Swallow DM, et al. Vascular disease and vascular risk factors in relation to motor features and cognition in early Parkinson's disease. Movement Disorders. 2016;**31**(10):1518-1526. DOI: 10.1002/mds.26698

[97] Gray MT, Woulfe JM. Striatal blood-brain barrier permeability in Parkinson's disease. Journal of Cerebral Blood Flow and Metabolism. 2015;**35**(5):747-750. DOI: 10.1038/jcbfm.2015.32

[98] Chung YC, Kim Y-S, Bok E, Yune TY, Maeng S, Jin BK. MMP-3 contributes to nigrostriatal dopaminergic neuronal loss, BBB damage, and neuroinflammation in an MPTP mouse model of Parkinson's disease. Mediators Inflamm. 2013; 370526. doi:10. 1155/2013/370526.

[99] Peelaerts W, Bousset L, Van der Perren A, Moskalyuk A, Pulizzi R, Giugliano M, Van den Haute C, Melki R, Baekelandt V. Synuclein strains cause distinct synucleinopathies after local and systemic administration. Nature. 2015; 522: 340-344. doi:10. 1038/nature14547.

[100] Sui Y-T, Bullock KM, Erickson MA, Zhang J, Banks WA. Alpha synuclein is transported into and out of the brain by the blood-brain barrier. Peptides. 2014;**62**:197-202. DOI: 10.1016/j.peptides.2014.09.018

[101] Vos CM, Geurts JJ, Montagne L, van Haastert ES, Bö L, van der Valk P, et al. Blood-brain barrier alterations in both focal and diffuse abnormalities on postmortem MRI in multiple sclerosis. Neurobiology of Disease. 2005;**20**(3):953-960. DOI: 10.1016/j.nbd.2005.06.012

[102] Alvarez JI, Cayrol R, Prat A. Disruption of central nervous system barriers in multiple sclerosis. Biochimica

et Biophysica Acta. 2011;**1812**(2):252-264. DOI: 10.1016/j.bbadis.2010.06.017

[103] Spencer JI, Bell JS, DeLuca GC. Vascular pathology in multiple sclerosis: reframing pathogenesis around the blood-brain barrier. Journal of Neurology, Neurosurgery, and Psychiatry. 2018;**89**(1):42-52. DOI: 10.1136/jnnp-2017-316011

[104] D'haeseleer M, Beelen R, Fierens Y, Cambron M, Vanbinst AM, Verborgh C, et al. Cerebral hypoperfusion in multiple sclerosis is reversible and mediated by endothelin-1. Proceedings of the National Academy of Sciences of the United States of America. 2013;**110**(14):5654-5658. DOI: 10.1073/pnas.1222560110

[105] Keep RF, Zhou N, Xiang J, Andjelkovic AV, Hua Y, Xi G. Vascular disruption and blood-brain barrier dysfunction in intracerebral hemorrhage. Fluids Barriers CNS. 2014;**11**:18. DOI: 10.1186/2045-8118-11-18

Chapter 3

Physical and Cognitive Therapy (PCT) in Critically Ill Patient

Heru Suwardianto

Abstract

The condition of Critically ill patients in the Intensive Care Unit (ICU) can make heavier impairment physical and cognitive functions. The research objective is to prove that physical-cognitive therapy affects towards increasing physical and cognitive functions to Critically ill patients in ICU. The research design was a Randomized Controlled Trials (RCTs). The samples were Critically ill patients in the ICU of Kediri Baptist Hospital as many as 64 Critically ill patients according to inclusion and exclusion criteria. The research has got ethical clearance from the Committee Ethics Medical Faculty of Diponegoro University. The research instrument used Physical Function ICU Test (PFIT) Indonesian Version and Mini-Mental State Examination (MMSE) Indonesian Version. The differential test used Independent t-test on physical function and Mann-Whitney test on cognitive function towards the intervention group and control group. The results showed that physical-cognitive therapy significantly affected increasing physical function ($P < 0.001$) with a mean increase of 3.2 points and cognitive function ($P < 0.001$) with a mean increase of 7.3 points. The difference test of influence between the intervention group and the control group was done by testing the posttest data on physical function ($P < 0.001$) and cognitive function ($P < 0.001$) in both groups. Effect size >0.8 (Physical Function: 3.2; Cognitive Function: 1.9). In conclusion, there was affecting physical-cognitive therapy towards increasing physical and cognitive functions to Critically ill patients in ICU.

Keywords: critically ill patient, intensive care unit, physical-cognitive therapy, physical function, mental stage

1. Introduction

1.1 Background

Critically ill patients with impaired physical function have a picture of the weakness of muscle quadriceps femoris, decreased strength, and decrease in daily activities. Critically ill patients will experience mechanical unloading and decreased neuromuscular activity. Patients critical during Intensive Care Unit (ICU) will lose 20% of muscle volume, and 70% of protein for 1 week are admitted to ICU. The study also found 476.862 patients (60% -80% of the total Critically ill patients in ICU with 30% of them unable to return to work (nonproductive) due to loss of muscle strength of 1% -2% each day after patient out of ICU [1–13]. Critically ill patients with decreased physical and cognitive functioning are caused by various treatment measures and the accompanying illness. Patients with physical and cognitive impairment were caused by a history of using a mechanical ventilator (33%), infection or sepsis (50%), patients receiving treatment 2 days up to >1 week in ICU (> 50%), delirium and critical illness or sepsis (70%), coronary heart disease (CHD) (36.6%), Unstable Angina (UA) (41.5%), Hypertension (19.5%), Supraventricular Tachycardia (SVT) (2.4%) [1, 2, 14, 15]. The main causal factors causing it are long-term care (≥2 days) and minimal mobilization. Other causative factors include previous medical history (health status and previous disease history), acute illness, critical illness (delirium, hypoxia, hypotension, glucose dysregulation, respiratory failure, shock, Congestive Heart Failure (CHF), sepsis and others), severity diseases, inflammation, loss of muscle strength, sedation, and anxiety levels (communication dissatisfaction, sleep disturbances) [4, 7, 9, 16, 17]. The critically ill patient decline in physical and cognitive functioning if not promptly prevented during ICU treatment may have an impact on increasing health problems when treated in the ICU and when out of the ICU. Critically ill patients with reduced physical and cognitive functioning if not promptly prevented during ICU may have the effect of aggravating and weakening the function of other organs.

Critical illness is associate with impaired brain function like cognitive impairment and mental health [9]. Brain function will reduce and patients in ICU will be Delirium. Neurotransmitters involved in delirium. There are a number of neurotransmitters believed to be involved in the pathogenesis of delirium, including acetylcholine, serotonin, dopamine, and gamma-aminobutyric acid (GABA) [18]. Peripheral inflammation (due to infection, surgery, or trauma) can induce brain parenchyma cells to release inflammatory cytokines. As a result, neurons and synapses dysfunction. In delirium patients, elevated levels of C-Reactive Protein (CRP), Interleukin-6 (IL-6), Tumor Necrois Factor alpha (TNF-α), Interleukin 1 Reseptor Antagonist (IL – 1RA), Interleukin-10 (IL-10), and Interleukin-8 (IL-8) were found. Critically ill patients may experience hemodynamic disturbances, blood pressure, heart rate, and other heart and brain conditions. This can worsen the critical condition of the patient while in the ICU.

Critically ill patients with decreased physical function were a condition that often arose. Which is characterized by a decrease in muscle and functional function [19]. Critically ill patients with decreased function can experience muscle atrophy which is caused by many factors, including inflammatory processes and responses, immobilization, nutritional deficiencies, administration of corticosteroids, and so on. Critically ill patients with impaired physical function have a picture of weakness in the musculus quadriceps femoris, decreased strength, and decreased in carrying out daily activities. Critically ill patients will experience mechanical unloading and decreased activity neuromuscular. Critically ill patients who experience decreased activity neuromuscular at a later stage experience stimulation of a complex adaptation response by producing a mechanism process protein synthesis, increased protein degradation, and increased apoptosis of muscle cells which are major contributors to muscle atrophy, decreased or lost muscle strength in patients.

Critically ill patients with decreased cognitive function can be described as a decrease in memory function and brain function, attention, executive function, mental processing speed visuospatial ability. Critically ill patients with decreased cognitive function are caused by a lack of knowledge about ICU care, ICU delirium, sedation, sleep disturbances, and hypoxia [3]. Critically ill patients with decreased cognitive function are associated with decreased brain oxidative metabolism that causes changes in regional neurotransmitters in the brain. Prefrontal and subcortical or there is a decrease in cholinergic and increased dopaminergic activity when the levels of serotonin and levels of GABA (Gamma-Aminobutyric Acid) are significant. The results of the study found that patients with decreased cognitive function occurred in 24% -34% of critically ill patients and were similar to the symptoms of traumatic brain injury (34%) and patients were similar to Alzheimer's disease and delirium (24%) [3–6, 8–11]. Decreased physical function can have an impact on weakness in other functions and reduce the quality of life of Critically ill patients.

Critically ill patients with decreased physical and cognitive function caused by various treatment measures and also the accompanying diseases. Critically ill patients with decreased physical and cognitive function due to a history of using mechanical ventilators (33%), infection or sepsis (50%), patients receiving 2 days to >1 week in ICU (> 50%), delirium and various critical illnesses or sepsis (70%), coronary heart disease (CHD) (36.6%), Unstable Angina (UA) (41.5%), Hypertension (19.5%), Supraventricular Tachycardia (SVT) (2,4%) [2, 14, 20, 21]. The main contributing factors that cause it are prolonged care (≥2 days) and minimal mobilization. Other contributing factors are previous medical history (health status and previous medical history), acute illness, critical illness (delirium, hypoxia, hypotension, glucose dysregulation, respiratory failure, shock, CHF (Congestive Heart Failure), sepsis. and others), disease severity, inflammation, loss of muscle strength, sedation, and anxiety levels (communication dissatisfaction, sleep disturbances) [4, 5, 22, 23]. Critically ill patients with decreased physical and cognitive function if not immediately prevented during ICU treatment can have an impact on increasing health problems while being admitted to the ICU and when leaving the ICU.

Critically ill patients with physical and cognitive decline if not prevented immediately while in the ICU, it can have an impact in the form of worsening and weakening the function of other organs [24]. Critically ill patients with decreased physical and cognitive function can have an impact on prolonged treatment time, decreased cognitive function, physical function (organs, muscle contractility, functional capacity and pain, vitality, fatigue) that persist, and worsening mental health (anxiety), emotional response, depression, reflection, loneliness, disability doing activities and using instruments in everyday life [4, 9, 23, 25–27]. Critically ill patients with the phenomenon of decreased physical and cognitive function based on the accompanying impact indicate the need for strategi preventive interventions while the patient is in the ICU. Function improvement in critically ill patients in the ICU increases with interventions given to each problem patient in the ICU and post ICU [3, 10, 20, 26, 28, 29].

1.2 Critical patient health problems

Problems of Critically ill Patients in the ICU is a health problem in the form of physical to psychological disorders that often appear and persist for a long time in patients who are through critical conditions in the ICU or when the patient is discharged from the ICU. The problem can be described as a collection of symptoms or an acute condition worsening the status of weakness in physical, cognitive, or mental health functions in the form of anxiety (physical, cognitive, and mental health) during critical illness. is a collection of symptoms from the patient's experience after the patient survives or is out of a critical period and/or at least ≥2 days in the ICU [4, 30, 31]. Problems during treatment in the ICU can be concluded in the form of a collection of symptoms shown in patients who have successfully passed critical conditions. From ICU and 3 symptoms or areas of damage shown, namely physical function impairment, cognitive impairment in the form of impaired orientation, registration, attention, calculation and language, and mental health impairment.

Causes of various patient problems while being treated until the patient is discharged from the ICU are Critically ill patients who have successfully passed their

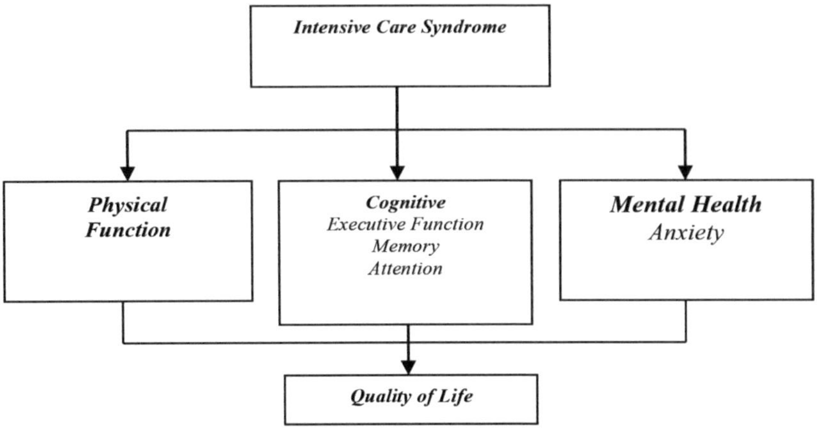

Figure 1.
Intensive care syndrome problems.

critical condition, being treated in the ICU ≥2 days with experiences that respond to patients [4]. A collection of symptoms of problems in the ICU can appear until the patient out of the ICU and the patient after being discharged from the hospital. Other causes include Critically ill patients who are treated in the ICU for a minimum period of 2 days with minimal mobilization, acute disease conditions, sepsis, and delirium. The impact is increasing the length of treatment time, mental health damage in the form of anxiety, physical function, and cognitive function [4, 10]. Critically ill patients with prolonged immobilization have an impact on physical function during the patient's stay in the ICU and after discharge from the ICU. These effects result in decreased organ function and decreased muscle contractility, functional capacity, and quality of life for patients [26]. Other causes based on the research include patients experiencing these problems, including Critically ill patients with acute illness, heart failure, Congestive Heart Failure (CHF), patients with sepsis, delirium, shock, etc. [3]. The results of research on Critically ill patients in the ICU found that 60% -80% of patients have functionally impaired, 50–70% patients have cognitively impaired (executive function, memory, and attention), and 10–40% of patients have experienced health deficits (anxiety, depression, and posttraumatic stress disorder (PTSD)) [3]. The magnitude of the impact that patients get after receiving treatment in the ICU can disrupt and reduce the patient's quality of life. Critically ill patients who are admitted to the ICU experience a decrease in muscle strength by 1–2% every day [10]. This can weaken physical function in the form of disuse atrophy, weakness in daily activities caused by immobilization or bed rest, ICU acquired illnesses, and age [3, 5, 32]. Post Intensive Care Syndrome (PICS) patients with the impaired physical function will interfere with life and health activities in patients in the form of productivity, activity daily, to the patient's quality of life. Symptoms in the ICU include physical impairment, cognitive impairment, and mental health in the form of degrees of anxiety (**Figure 1**).

2. Cognitive and physical impairment

2.1 Cognitive impairment

The results of post ICU patient research can cause cognitive impairment, with severity 34% of patients have damage cognitive impairment is similar to traumatic brain injury, and 24% of patients have cognitive impairment similar to Alzheimer's disease, and delirium, which is a separate risk factor for long-term cognitive impairment [8]. The study of 637,867 patients who survived the ICU from 1999 to 2008 showed that patients experience cognitive impairment and functional and is increasing significantly [4].

The results investigations Pre and post ICU found that the prevalence of cognitive impairment increased from initially moderate to a more severe scale with an increase in the value of 6.1% [6]. Cognitive impairment in Critically ill patients who are treated in the ICU can have manifestations of acute brain dysfunction to delirium. Delirium is characteristic of changes in mental status and fluctuating course [24]. Long-standing cognitive impairment can lead to cognitive deficits by following the severity of the pain, which in turn worsens and weakens other functions [24]. Decreased cognitive function is also associated with decreased brain oxidative metabolism causing neurotransmitter changes in the prefrontal and subcortical areas. There was a decrease in cholinergic activity and an increase in dopaminergic activity, at a time when the significance of serotonin and GABA levels remained unclear.

2.1.1 Measurement of cognitive function of patients in the ICU

1. Questionnaire on Cognitive Decline in The Elderly (IQCODE)

Critically ill patients have a form of cognitive dysfunction in the long term that still needs further research. This cognitive dysfunction is characterized by pre-existing mild exacerbation deficits, global and executive cognitive function. Long-term cognitive impairment after a patient can pass through a critical illness can become a new problem and reduce the quality of life. The results of the study found that the cognitive function of Critically ill patients can be measured using the Questionnaire on Cognitive Decline in The Elderly (IQCODE). Questionnaire on Cognitive Decline in The Elderly (IQCODE) has 26 question items that have good correlation, test–retest reliabilities [33]. This instrument can also be given to dementia patients, the results of other studies also show that Questionnaire on Cognitive Decline in The Elderly (IQCODE) has high reliability.

2. The Mini-Mental State Examination (MMSE)

Measurement of a patient's cognitive status uses the mini-mental state examination (MMSE). The mini-mental state examination is a tool to measure mental status which in this case is cognitive impairment. The mini-mental state examination is a measuring tool that has high reliability and validity so that it can describe cognitive functions. The mini-mental state examination has 11 questions in which there are five areas of cognitive function, namely orientation, registration, attention, and calculation, recall, and language the maximum score is 30. Scores of 23 and below indicates cognitive impairment. Long duration measurement The mini-mental state examination (MMSE) for 5–10 minutes [34].

2.2 Physical impairment

Critically ill patients in the ICU during bed rest will experience mechanical unloading and decreased activity neuromuscular, which in turn stimulates a complex adaptation response by showing protein synthesis, increased protein degradation, and increased apoptosis of muscle cells. This mechanism is a major contributor to muscle atrophy and decreased or loss of muscle strength in patients, it can be seen after the patient's bed rest. Muscle metabolism disorders that occur

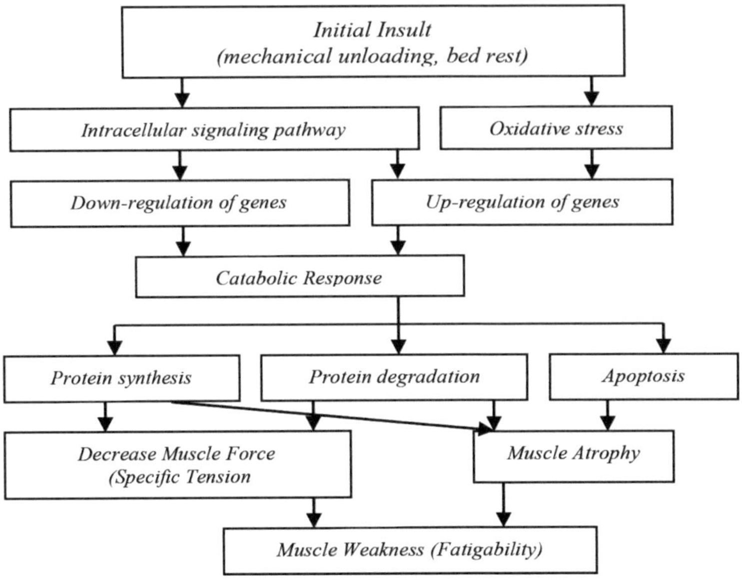

Figure 2.
The immobilization-induced catabolic response.

reduce protein formation to energy breakdown during patient immobilization or bed rest.

Critically ill patients in the ICU show that 70% of the minimum activity will lose muscle mass after bed rest, especially in the lower extremities [19]. The results of a study on Critically ill patients who were treated in the ICU with a research method using RCTs (Randomized Controlled Trials) found that patients who hospitalized in the ICU > 48 hours will experience impaired physical function and sleep disturbances [35]. Critically ill patients in the ICU with minimal mobilization, disease prognosis, unusual environment, and sedation response affect the patient's comfort response and affect the response of the hormone oxytocin.

A decrease in the quality of sleep of a critical patient will increase the patient's anxiety so that the patient is unable to be oriented and cooperative. Physical response muscle weakness can increase the discomfort response so that the patient's body is in a state of oxidative stress. Oxidative stress occurs because several free radicals in the body exceed the body's capacity to neutralize them. The impact of this is that the intensity of the oxidation process in normal body cells becomes higher and causes significant and more damage. Oxidative stress is the main cause, one of which is the emergence of chronic diseases such as cancer, heart disease, Alzheimer's, and others (**Figure 2**).

2.2.1 Measurement of physical function of critically ill patients in the ICU

Measurement of physical function can be done with several measuring instruments including Time up and Go (TUG) Test

a. Time Up and Go [36]

TUG is a physical function measuring tool by assessing balance and the risk of falling. The tools used are a stopwatch, a chair, a meter with a minimum length of 3 meters, or 10 feet. The patient is instructed by the nurse and the patient must follow suit. The patient performs mobilization from sitting to standing and walking. The interpretation of Time up and Go (TUG) is the time taken from sitting to standing.

Interpretation of ≤ 10 seconds is normal, ≤ 20 seconds is good mobilization, can walk alone, mobilize without the aid of tools, ≤ 30 seconds is a problem, cannot go independently, requires tool assistance, ≥ 14 seconds the patient has a high risk of falling.

b. 6 Minute Walk Test (MWT)

Physical function measurement with instruments 6 Minute Test (6 MWT) to measure the patient's physical functioning endurance. The tools needed for this measurement are a stopwatch, rolling tape, aisle. The measurement carried out is the distance the patient has walked for 6 minutes [37]. The measurement is stopped if it finds the following criteria, signs, and symptoms of angina (chest pain), dizziness, confusion, ataxia, staggering, unsteadiness, pallor, cyanosis, nausea, dyspnea, fatigue, signs of peripheral circulatory insufficiency, claudication or significant pain, and the patient develops distress. Discontinue if there are hemodynamic changes such as systolic blood pressure decreases >10 mmHg, systolic blood pressure increases >250 mmHg, diastolic blood pressure rises >120 mmHg, and HR falls >15 beats per minute.

c. Physical Function ICU Test (PFIT)

The physical strength of patients in the ICU is usually measured by looking at the patient's ability to perform or meet the needs of daily activities. The physical function of a critical patient can be measured to determine the degree of physical function impairment in the patient. Examination or measurement of physical function is expected to be able to present the real condition of the critical patient's condition in the ICU or after the patient is discharged from the ICU. physical in the ICU are responsibility, reliability and validity can use Physical Function ICU Test (PFIT). Physical Function ICU Test (PFIT) is a physical function measurement tool that can be used by critical nurses in the ICU to identify the condition of critically ill patients in the ICU. The Physical Function ICU Test is proven to be safe with high clinical utility, responsiveness to all changes, and PFIT is recommended in testing the physical function of patients in the ICU [38–40]. PFIT shows good reliability and responsiveness to changes and the respondents who take measurements safe and flexible [39]. The PFIT test was carried out on 20 respondents and all respondents measured the results obtained $P < 0.05$. The Physical Function ICU Test can show an increase in the progress of muscle function and muscle strength in Critically ill patients [39]. The Physical Function ICU Test can be performed on patients with a tracheostomy attached, a ventilator, the patient can follow orders, can sit, and not. Performed in patients with a fraction of inspired oxygen (Fio_2) > 0.6 (> 60%); positive end-expiratory pressure (PEEP) > 8 cmH_2O; patients with spinal cord injuries, stroke, and unstable fractures [39]. There are 4 Physical Function ICU Test (PFIT) domains measured, namely:

3. Physical-cognitive therapy

3.1 Definition

Early activity therapy intervention in the ICU is an effort to prevent the worsening of the patient's muscle condition or weakness after the patient is discharged from the ICU [41]. Cognitive therapy is therapy in Critically ill patients to reduce the possibility and insecurity of the patient while in the ICU. Due to decreased cognitive function [24]. Physical-cognitive therapy is a critical ICU patient intervention that allows cognitive and physical damage due to short or long bed rest [24]. Based on the results of the study showed that cognitive therapy was effective in improving cognitive function in ICU patients.

Physical-cognitive therapy-pharmacological is a nonprevention and management to improve cognitive quality and physical function (Miller and Ely, 2007) intervention physical-cognitive therapy can improve the cognitive and physical function of Critically ill patients in the ICU and after the patient leaves the ICU. Therapy is given for no more than 20 minutes due to the response fatigue patients during ICU treatment and the response to hemodynamic changes during fatigue.

Physical and cognitive exercise interventions are appropriate and recommended by the Nursing Interventions Classification (NIC). Physical exercise can be done by teaching exercise prescribing (5612), positioning (0840), neurological positioning (0844), increasing strength training (0201), stretching exercises (0202), improving body mechanics (0140), and rehabilitative cardiac care (4046). Cognitive exercise can be done with delusional management (6440) which supports the comfort and orientation to the reality of the patient [42].

3.2 Physical-cognitive therapy screening

Interventions Physical-cognitive therapy (PCT) is implemented to the patient once a day at ±10.00 a.m. because at that time it is the body's metabolic response in the best conditions. Intervention is carried out for a maximum of 20 minutes for 3 days according to the patient's condition or adjusted to the Richmond Agitation Sedation Scale (RASS) so that patients get intervention according to their needs and abilities because muscle and neurotransmitter metabolism can achieve maximum function if therapy is carried out continuously.

Physical-cognitive therapy can be performed in Critically ill patients with respiratory failure, patients on noninvasive ventilators pressure ventilation, high flow nasal cannula, shock (Dopamine ≥7.5 mcg/kg/min, Norepinephrine ≥5 mcg/kg/min, Dobutamine ≥5 mcg / kg / min, Phenylephrine ≥75 mcg/kg/min, Epinephrine, Vasopressin >0.03 mcg/min). This intervention should be avoided in patients >72 hours after the development of respiratory failure or shock, cardiac surgery, and post-cardiac arrest. This intervention is only given a maximum of 20 minutes [24].

The first intervention procedure physical-cognitive therapy, namely Critically ill patients in the ICU, is first assessed by RASS. Patients with RASS score of -5 to −4 and − 3 to −2, started to physical therapy intervention using passive Range of Motion (ROM). Patients with RASS score of −3 to −2 patients started to learn cognitive training in the form of space, place, time, and people orientation. The patients with RASS score of −1, 0, +1, would start for physical exercise in the form of active exercise, including sitting beside the bed, standing or moving, Activity Daily Living (ADL) training such as eating, drinking, eliminating, changing positions and finally walking. Meanwhile, for the patient's cognitive training, orientation training Interventions were carried out, digit span forward, matrix puzzle, digit span reverse, noun list recall, paragraph or story recall, letter-number sequences, pattern recognition. Patients with RASS score of −3 to −2 started to learn cognitive training in the form of space, place, time, and people orientation. The patients with RASS score of −1, 0, +1 would start physical exercise in the form of active exercise, including sitting beside the bed, standing or moving, training of Activity Daily Living (ADL) such as eating, drinking, eliminating, changing positions, and finally walking.

3.3 Intervention procedures cognitive therapy

Intervention therapy Cognitive is a cognitive exercise given to patients for a maximum of 20 minutes for 1 time a day for at least 3 days of implementation.

Before implementing the intervention, an assessment of the patient's level of consciousness was carried out using RASS. The goal intervention cognitive therapy is to increase or prevent cognitive decline during treatment in the ICU or after being discharged from the ICU. The patient was not intervened if the patient was stupors or comatose (RASS -4 to −5). The patient was able to respond to sound but was unable to maintain it (awake) or maintain eye contact for >10 seconds (RASS -3 to −2), then the patient was subjected to orientation training intervention. A series of exercises given to the patient's alert (RASS -1 to +1). The patient is subjected to cognitive stimulation from orientation exercises to the stages for a maximum of 20 minutes. Patients are given Interventions to the extent that the patient achieves them within a time limit of 20 minutes [24, 29].

1. Orientation Exercises

Patients are asked to answer 10 orientation questions and are assessed. Five questions are questions related to time orientation (current year, season, month, date, and day). The next five questions assessed the orientation of the place including city, state, province, where the patient is (ICU hospital), and what floor the patient is currently hospitalized for. The orientation of time and place is instantaneous. Correctly answered questions were repeated starting over for all or 10 orientation questions.

2. Digit Span-Forward

The patient is asked to repeat a sequence of numbers, starting with a 4-digit sequence (for example, 4–1–2-8) and advancing to a 9-digit sequence (for example, 6–1–4 – 2-9- 3- 5-7-8).

3. Matrix Puzzle

Patients are asked to choose the correct answer from a series of five answers that complete a matrix pattern.

4. Digit Span Reverse

Similar to "Digit Span-Forward" above, the patient is asked to repeat the sequence in reverse order. For example, suppose the patient is given the sequence 5–7 – 3, and the patient is asked to repeat it in the reverse order, "3–7-5". Exercises start with a 3-sequence digit and progress to an 8-sequence digit.

5. Noun List Recall

The patient reads a series of seven words and is asked to repeat them in any order, for example, "cat, cat, clock, foot, guitar, knife, button".

6. Paragraph or Story Recall

Patients read a story that contains many details and are asked to repeat it back to the nurse or researcher as they have read. For example, "On March 14, two cows escaped from their pen through a hole in the fence and went to a busy highway, three cars collided trying to avoid the cow, fortunately, no one was injured. After four hours the cow just went down. can be caught".

7. Letter-Number Sequences

Patients are asked to read a sequence of letters and numbers after which they are asked to arrange letters and numbers and the numerical sequence is first ordered then alphabetical order. This exercise starts with a series of 1 number and letters (for example, "L, 2", and the patient will answer, "2-L") and progresses to 4 numbers and 4 letters (for example, "7, M, 2, T, 6, F, 1, Z", to which the patient will answer "1–2–6-7-FMTZ").

8. Pattern Recognition

The patient is presented with a sequence of letters or numbers with some of the sequences omitted. The patient is then asked to complete the sequence by recognizing the pattern of the components. Which is missing and fills in the missing letters or numbers (for example, the sequence: 1 -__- 3 - __ - 5 - __ - 7 - __ will finish by filling in the missing even numbers, 1–2 - 3 - 4 - 5 - 6 - 7 - 8).

3.4 Intervention procedures physical therapy

Physical therapy is physical activity therapy carried out on Critically ill patients in the ICU by paying attention to the patient's condition with the hope of improving the patient's physical function recovery. The goal of physical therapy is to improve the patient's physical function while the patient is in the ICU contractures, or atrophy during the patient's life emphasizes the treatment and, in the end, the patient's physical function after leaving the ICU is getting better. is a physical activity therapy performed on Critically ill patients in the ICU by paying attention to the patient's condition with the hope of improving the recovery of the patient's physical function. Intervention physical therapy Before, necessary screening is.

Criteria Patients who receive physical exercise interventions have the following signs and symptoms 43:

1. Decreased pulse pressure (e.g., lightheadedness and syncope).

2. Heart rate is 40 to 130 beats/minute

3. Respiratory rate is 5 to 40 breaths/minute.

4. Systolic blood pressure > 180 mmHg.

5. Pulse oximetry <88%.

6. Marked ventilator desynchrony.

7. Patient distress (nonverbal cues, gestures, physical combativeness).

The intervention was immediately stopped, the patient was instructed in a resting position (for example, sitting in a chair, on the edge of the bed or supine on the bed), but if the intervention was able to be completed within 5 minutes, the next intervention was based on the clinical judgment from the intervention provider or the therapist. If the patient presents with an arrhythmia, or if there is any concern that new myocardial ischemia, impaired breathing and airway patterns of the patient, or if the patient has fallen, then the intervention is stopped immediately. If the patient is found to have a change in the RASS value to +2, +3, or + 4, the procedure is immediately stopped. If there is a change in the RASS value on a different day, then the therapy is stopped (drop out) Physical exercise procedures, namely:

1. Patients in a coma or stupor (RASS −4 or − 5): passive ROM intervention is performed (Abduction of the shoulder, elbow, and groin. Knee extension., flexion and dorsiflexion of the ankle).

2. Patients with RASS -3 or − 2: passive ROM intervention was performed and the patient was positioned to sit in bed for at least 20 minutes.

3. Patients with RASS -1 to 1: identified as capable of active ROM, then the patient performs active ROM in all major joints and/or sleep mobility exercises (for example, lateral and supine tilts and sitting), sitting on the edge of the bed, doing daily activities -day (eating or simulating eating, bathing or brushing teeth, dressing), changing positions from sitting to standing and from bed to chair, and ambulation (with or without assistance).

Measurement of physical and cognitive function outcomes can be done 72 hours after the intervention or the patient is discharged from the ICU [24].

4. Theory the symptom management

Symptom management model first was introduced at the University of California, San Francisco (UCSF) by Larson in 1994, and developed by Dodd, M., Janson, S., Facione, N., Faucett, J., Froelicher, ES, Humphreys, J., Taylor, D. in 2001 in the publication of the Journal of Advanced Nursing with the title Advancing the Science of Symptom Management. (Dodd et al., 2001) Symptoms are defined as subjective experiences that reflect changes in the biopsychosocial function, sensation, or cognition of the individual. Signs and symptoms are defined as disease indications detected by individuals or other people. (Smith & Liehr, 2014) Signs and symptoms of problems are in the form of cognitive and physical dysfunction, which are important aspects of health status and diseases that interfere with the health of other patients such as social function. Acute symptoms that often appear will make patients come back to health services to have their health checked and make the patient's quality of life decrease (**Figure 3**).

Patients during treatment in the ICU may develop symptoms or a group of symptoms that can be the first indication in identifying the prognosis of further disease progression. These symptoms are the effect of previous treatment while in the ICU or symptoms of decreased health function can also be caused by pharmacologists or nursing services performed by health personnel. Theory of Symptom Management can help provide information to relieve or prevent symptoms or to minimize the stress of experiencing symptoms that can occur while a patient is in the ICU. This middle-range theory serves to guide symptom assessment and Interventions in nursing practice [20, 43].

Three important concepts of Symptom Management Theory (SMT) namely, symptom experience, symptom management strategies, and symptom status outcomes. This concept focuses on three domains of nursing science, namely the domain of people, environment, and health or disease (person domain, environmental domain, and health/illness domain) as contextual considerations for nursing research [43].

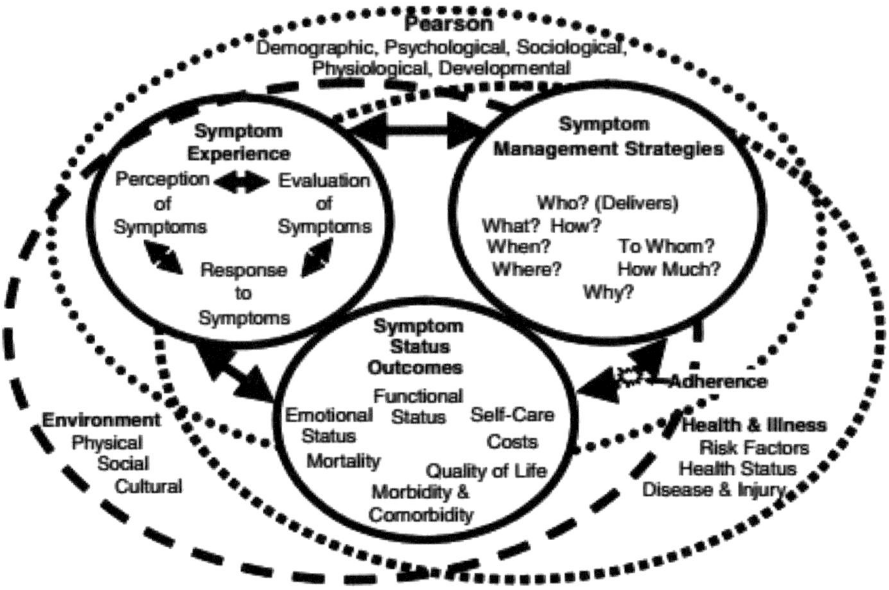

Figure 3.
Symptom management [44].

Critical patients in the ICU will have various illness symtoms, depending on age and reproductive status as well as other factors. These factors include genetic risk factors (person domain), cultural beliefs, the representative meaning of a symptom based on reported laboratory and the diagnosis of the disease (health or disease domain). Experience history of pain while in the ICU is a simultaneous perception, evaluation, and response to changes in a person. Changes can be identified how often (frequency) the condition is sick or how severe (how bad) the condition or illness is. The frequency or severity may not change, but the stress associated with symptom problems in the ICU can be altered by preventive intervention strategies. Symptomatic experiences can include not one but several synergistic symptoms. Strategies Symptom management to prevent, delay, or minimize the experience of symptoms of patient problems while in the ICU should be applicable. This strategy can be effective in three ways: (1) reducing the frequency of symptom experiences, (2) minimizing symptom severity, or (3) eliminating the pain associated with symptoms (**Figure 3**) [44].

5. Result

In this work, our objective is to prove that physical-cognitive therapy (PCT) affects towards increasing physical and cognitive functions to critical patients in ICU with design was Randomized Controlled Trials (RCTs). This research data was obtained by determining the criteria for respondents. The Inclusion criteria include Patients who have been treated in ICU ≥ 24 hours, RASS -5 to +1, No visual disturbance, and hearing. Exclusion criteria include RASS +2, +3, and + 4, Patients who change RASS values to +2, +3 and + 4 when intervened or different days, Patients screening scores change during intervention, Patient forcibly return home or refer to another hospital, Patient dies, Initial assessment or ongoing intervention in patients is found with Cardiac Surgery, Neurodegenerative

No	Characteristic	Group		Z	P-Value (N = 64)
		Intervention (N = 32)	Control (N = 32)		
1	**Gender**				
	Male	19 (59.4%)	16 (50%)	0.74	0.455
	Female	13 (40.6%)	16 (50%)		
2	**Age** ($\bar{x}$ ± SD)	59.9 ± 10.94	48.03 ± 11.4		<0.001
	12–16-Year-old	—	1 (3.1%)	3.78	
	26–35-Year-old	—	2 (6.4%)		
	36–45-Year-old	4 (12.5%)	10 (31.3%)		
	46–55-Year-old	7 (21.9%)	11 (34.4%)		
	56–65-Year-old	11 (34.4%)	7 (21.9%)		
	> 65-Year-old	10 (31.3%)	1 (3.1%)		
3	**Diagnose**				
	CHD -UA	5 (15.6%)	10 (31.3%)	1.01	0.312
	CHD- OMI	11 (34.4%)	7 (21.9%)		
	decomp cordis phase class III-IV	7 (21.9%)	7 (21.9%)		
	HHF	3 (9.4%)	3 (9.4%)		
	Pneumothorax	2 (6.3%)	—		
	Acidosis metabolic	1 (3.1%)	—		
	DKA	1 (3.1%)	—		
	COPD	1 (3.1%)	—		
	Asthma Attack Emergency	1 (3.1%)	—		
	Observation Ileus	—	2 (6.3%)		
	Stroke Hemorrhagic	—	1 (3.1%)		
	GEA	—	1 (3.1%)		
	Hyperglycemic	—	1 (3.1%)		
4	**RASS**				
	+1	1 (3.1%)	3 (9.4%)	2.06	0.039
	0	16 (50.0%)	19 (59.4%)		
	-1	—	4 (12.5%)		
	-2	10 (31.3%)	6 (18.8%)		
	-3	4 (12.5%)	—		
	-4	1 (3.1%)	—		
5	**Sedation**				
	Yes	23 (71.9%)	22 (68.8%)	3.07	0.002
	No	9 (28.1%)	10 (28.1%)		

Notes: [a]*: Chi-Square test,* [b]*: Mann- Whitney test; Z: Z count (Z table: 1.96); CHD: Coronary Heart Disease; UA: unstable angina; OMI: old myocardia infarct; HHF: Hypertension heart failure; DKA: diabetic ketoacidosis; COPD: chronic obstructive Pulmonary Disease; GEA: gastroenteritis acute.*

Table 1.
Respondent characteristic.

Group	Mean Rank	Sum Rank	U	P-value
Physical Function			13.00	<0.001
Intervention	48.09	1539.00		
Control	16.91	541.00		

Table 2.
Differences of physical function test results between intervention group and critical patient control group (N = 64).

disease, Post cardiac arrest with suspected anoxic brain injury, Unstable fracture, long bones and open abdomen, Psychotic disorder. The population in the study were all critical patients treated at Kediri Baptist Hospital. Based on ICU RS. Baptist Kediri in May–June 2017 there were 267 patients treated in ICU. The samples were critical patients in ICU of Baptist Hospital Kediri as many as 64 critical patients according to inclusion and exclusion criteria. Independent variable in this research is physical-cognitive therapy. Dependent variable in this research is physical function and cognitive function. The research tool in this research is physical function measurement tool (PFIT) and cognitive function. Data collection has been done after completing the research proposal. Researcher get ethical clearance from KEPK Medical Faculty of Diponegoro University, and Researcher apply research permission from Diponegoro University Semarang to Director of RS. Baptist Kediri. The Wilcoxon test was used to determine differences in cognitive-physical function before and after physical cognitive therapy in each group, whereas the Mann Whitney test was used to determine the posttest of cognitive-physical function between the intervention group and the control group. The value of confidence interval applied is 95% with significance level 5% ($\alpha = 0.05$). The data obtained is used to support the discussion regarding factors that can affect the research variables.

The characteristic information of subjects is listed in **Table 1**. There were slightly gender differences in the two groups; including more than 50% male in the intervention group while balanced amount between male and female sex in the control group. The subjects of the study in both groups had an average adult age to the early elderly. Diagnosis symptoms varied in the two groups; for example, less than 50% (34.4%) had diagnoses of OMI CHD for the intervention group of the research subjects, while only 21.9% in the control group. More than 50% Research subjects in the two groups had a calm and alert awareness level of 0 (RASS = 0). Majority subjects received sedation in the intervention group (71.9%) and the control group (64%) (**Table 1**).

The result of the test result is the mean rank of the control group is 16.91 and the intervention group is 48.09, with each sum rank is 1539.00 and 541.00. The mean rank result is known that the physical function in the intervention group is better than the control group. The value of U arithmetic is ($13 < 105$) with the significance of P-value (<0.001), indicating that there was a significant influence difference in the physical function between the intervention group and the control group (**Table 2**).

The result of the test result is the control group's mean rank is 19.28 and the intervention group is 45.72, with each sum rank is 1463.00 and 612.00. The mean rank result is known that cognitive function in the intervention group is better than the control group. The value of U arithmetic is ($13 < 105$) with significance P-value (<0.001), which means that there is a significant effect difference in the cognitive function between the intervention group and the control group (**Table 3**).

Group	Mean Rank	Sum Rank	U	P-value
Cognitive Function			89.00	<0.001
Intervention	45.72	1463.00		
Control	19.28	617.00		

Table 3.
Results of differences in cognitive function assessment of intervention groups and critical patient control groups (N = 64).

6. Discussion

Brain function will be impairment if there is not preventive intervention in ICU. Patients will get impairment cognitive, physical functional, delirium, impairment hormone in the brain. The brain will release oxidative stress, the body compensates by reducing oxidative metabolism in the brain. As a result, brain dysfunction occurs which causes delirium symptoms. This condition also triggers the formation of reactive oxygen and nitrogen which worsens the damage to brain tissue. This damage is permanent and causes complications in the form of permanent cognitive decline. Disturbance in Critically ill patients will also create an imbalance of neurotransmitters, especially acetylcholine and dopamine. Acetylcholine levels were found to be decreased in delirium patients in the ICU. These levels return to normal after the patient is no longer delirium. Additionally, anticholinergic drugs (acetylcholine blockers) have been shown to cause delirium. Dopamine and acetylcholine have a reciprocal (opposite) relationship. There is an increase in dopamine levels in delirium. The administration of dopamine blockers can also reduce symptoms of delirium. Serotonin is increased in hepatic encephalopathy and septic delirium. Serotonin agonists (hallucinogenic drugs) can also cause delirium. In critically ill patients with delirium, changes in gamma-aminobutyric acid (GABA) and histamine levels occur. Changes can be either increasing or decreasing, depending on the cause of the delirium. Neuroendocrine disorders can also occur where this hormone is associated with increased proinflammatory cytokines in the brain and neuronal damage. The neuroendocrine hypothesis also explains the development of delirium in patients receiving exogenous glucocorticoids. Circadian cycle disruption can affect sleep quality and physiology. Lack of sleep can lead to delirium, memory deficits, and psychosis. Melatonin is a hormone that regulates the circadian cycle. One study shows a link between low melatonin levels and the incidence of delirium. Another study says that administering exogenous melatonin to hospitalized patients reduces the incidence of delirium.

Physical Cognitive Therapy significantly affects physical function in critically ill patients in the ICU. The subjects of the study intervention group increased physical function after intervention with a mean difference of the increase in the intervention group of 3.2, whereas in the control group decreased physical function with a mean of 0.2. The intervention group increased physical function because of physical exercise that is done properly and regularly. Physical exercise at each joint can increase the activity of mechanisms neuromuscular Critically ill patients during bed rest. Physical activity done regularly prevents apoptosis activity. The control group decreased physical function due to a decrease in neuromuscular muscle-debilitating up until the occurrence of cell apoptosis. Improved physical function occurs along with increased functionality and functional use of aid mobilization, step, shoulder strength, and the strength of the knee. Physical-cognitive therapy is expected to be physiologically capable of activating mechanical neuromuscular patients, it is supported by the theory that in principle, the physical exercises to stimulate muscle nerves to recognize that when the patient bed rest does not happen mechanical unloading and decreased neuromuscular activity. The results of research supported by the theories Margaret that moment activity neuromuscular becomes better, it will inhibit the complex adaptation response (protein synthesis), protein degradation, and apoptosis of muscle cells [1, 2, 6, 7–13, 15, 21, 30, 31, 45–56]. Mechanisms that occur are the main contributor muscle atrophy, loss of muscle strength in critically ill patients during bed rest. Physical-cognitive therapy is expected to increase muscle metabolism which further increases the formation of protein to energy solution for patient immobilization or bed rest. Physical-Cognitive therapy can improve physical function declined over the patient in the ICU, it was supported by the results of research Thomsen stated that ambulation and early mobilization in critically ill patients in the ICU were able to improve the patient's physical function and also decrease the use of sedation [57]. Critically ill patients in ICU should be done as soon as possible physical mobility exercises to improve muscle metabolism and does not activate a response or apoptosis mechanism. The results of research supported by Elliott in the prevention of damage to physical function after discharge from the ICU who stated that early mobility can mitigate the negative impact of critical illness and improved its physical function [20].

Physical-cognitive therapy significantly impacts on improving the cognitive functions of Critically ill patients in ICU. These results correspond with the results of a study that critically ill patients in the ICU can experience mental health disorders such as anxiety and they have cognitive impairment and poor sleep quality.[5] Improved cognitive function was not affected by the characteristics of the study subjects from the intervention group. The decline in cognitive function is influenced also by gender by the statistical results and strengthened by the results of cognitive function decline Wreksoatmojo is motivated by a variety of risk factors that cannot be avoided such as age and gender, as well as some physical conditions and diseases [58]. The decline in cognitive function can slow recovery in patients. The research subjects in the control group were restless anxiety and pain scale settled on the first day to the third day.

The results also showed increased cognitive function occurred in all subdomains variable orientation, regression, attention-calculation, recall, and language. Research shows that physical-cognitive therapy can improve the function of any existing variables. The results of research supported by the results of studies that suggest that cognitive therapy can change the perception of self in patients with heart problems [59]. Research subjects most heart problems with a variety of conditions and consciousness and care in the ICU. The subjects of the study intervention group experienced an increase in all indicators of cognitive function. Cognitive function has several major functions in which work is recertified function, memory function, the function of thinking, and repressive function. This repressive function involves the ability to make the selection process, clarify and integrate the information provided. Researchers on the provision of physical-cognitive therapy provide the stimuli of orientation, registration, attention-calculation, recall until the language with the hope of the study subjects were able to do the selection process to integrate more complex information. The research subjects' control group decreased cognitive function have a significant relationship to independence by the results of research conducted by Balquis [60]. Subjects have been unable to carry out compliance activities of daily needs and also experience pain at a mild to moderate level. It also can affect the patient's condition, especially the condition of his illness. Based on the results that research subjects have the most control group cognitive impairment in moderate time in the ICU.

The research subjects in the control group with a decline in cognitive function may occur and demonstrate emotional response after discharge from the ICU such as anxiety, depression, fatigue, reflection, and solitude in accordance expressed by Strahan.[21] cognitive decline will worsen and weaken the function of other organs if not prevented in treatment in the ICU [29]. These results are also supported by another theory which states that the impact of the decline in cognitive function for patients in ICU that increase the treatment time, a decline in cognitive function, physical function (organs, muscle contractility, functional capacity and pain, vitality, fatigue), and worsening mental health (anxiety), emotional responses, depression, reflection, loneliness, inability to perform the activity and the use of instruments in everyday life. Condition of patients with worsening cognitive function for patients in ICU should be prevented to maintain the patient's quality of life and function as whole human beings with various functions in carrying out daily activities. Approach to symptom management theory indicated expected any problems can be overcome by a specific patient. Specific Nursing Interventions applied and overcome specific problems as well. The results also were able to study the possible factors that need to be improved in the provision of Interventions, to provide maximum benefit to patients on the signs and symptoms of health problems in critically ill patients in the ICU.

Acknowledgements

I would like to offer my special thanks to patients in ICU Kediri Baptist Hospital. I would like to thank dr. Jati Listiyanto Pujo, Sp. An., KIC., Erina Purwanti (intensivist), Dr. dr. Awal Prasetyo, Sp.THT-KL, M. Kes, and Ns. Reni Sulung Utami, S. Kep, MSc for their help in this research.

Author details

Heru Suwardianto
Baptist Hospital Health Collage, Kediri, Indonesia

*Address all correspondence to: herusuwardianto@gmail.com

References

[1] Davidson JE, Hopkins RO, Louis D, Iwarshyna T (2013) Post-intensive care syndrome. Soc Crit Care Med 1:1-4

[2] Iwashyna TJ (2014) Post-intensive care syndrome: improving the future of icu patients. 24nd Crit Care Congr Rev 1:13-16

[3] Needham DM, Davidson J, Cohen H, et al (2012) Improving long-term outcomes after discharge from intensive care unit: report from a stakeholders' conference. Crit Care Med 40:502-509

[4] Iwashyna T (2014) What you need to know about post-intensive care syndrome (PICS). Heal Syst Michigan 1:1-3

[5] Rahimi RA, Skrzat J, S. RDR, Zanni JM, Fan E, Stephens RS, Needhan DM (2013) Physical rehabilitation of patients in the intensive care unit requiring extracorporeal membrane oxygenation: a small case series. Phys Ther 93:248-255

[6] Iwashyna TJ, Cooke CR, Wunsch H, Kahm JM (2012) Population burden of long-term survivorship after severe sepsis in older americans. J Compil © 2012, Am Geriatr Soc 60:1070-1077

[7] Needham DM (2012) Improving long-term outcomes after discharge from intensive care unit: Report from a stakeholders' conference. Crit Care Med 40:502-509

[8] Pandharipande P, Girard T, Morandi A, Thompsom J (2013) Long-term cognitive impairment after critical illness. New Engl J Med 369:1306-1316

[9] Jackson J, Pandharipande P, Girard T, Brummed N, Thompson J (2014) Depression, post-traumatic stress disorder, and functional disability in survivors of critical illness in the brain-icu study: a longitudinal cohort study. Lancet Respir Med 2:369-379

[10] Sottile, Peter, Amy Nordon-Craft, Daniel Malone, Darcie M. Luby, Margaret Schenkman MM (2015) Physical therapis treatment of patients in the neurogical intensive care unit: description of practice. Phys Ther 95:1006-1014

[11] Cartwright MM (2012) The high incidence of post intensive care unit (ICU) anxiety and depression. Psychol Today 1

[12] Suwardianto H (2015) Buku ajar keperawatan kegawatdaruratan (perspektif, konsep, prinsip, dan penatalaksanaan kegawatdaruratan), 1st ed. PT. REVKA PETRA MEDIA, Surabaya

[13] Suwardianto H, Selvia D (2015) Buku Ajar Keperawatan Kegawatdaruratan (Perspektif, Konsep, Prinsip, dan Penatalaksanaan Kegawatdaruratan). PT. REVKA PETRA MEDIA, Surabaya

[14] Hoffman LA, Guttendorf J (2015) Post Intensive care syndrome: risk factors and prevention strategies. AHC media 1

[15] Suwardianto H (2016) Tardive dyskenesia, motor activity, sedation scale, and cardiac workload in baptis kediri hospital. World Soc Disaster Nurs 4:1

[16] Hopkins RO (2013) Strategies to ensure long-term quality of life in ICU survivors. Soc Crit Care Med 1:1

[17] Needham DM, Davidson J, Cohan H, PharmD, Hopkins R (2012) Improving long-term outcomes after discharge from intensive care unit: report from a stakeholders' conference.

Soc Crit Care Med Lippincott Williams Wilkins 40:502-509

[18] Ali S, Patel M, Jabeen S, Bailey RK, Patel T, Shahid M, Riley WJ, Arain A (2011) Insight into delirium. Innov Clin Neurosci 8:25-34

[19] Poulsen JB (2012) Impaired physical function, loss of muscle mass and assessment of biomechanical properties in critical ill patients. Dan. Med. J.

[20] Davidson JE, Harvey M a, Bemis-Dougherty A, Smith JM, Hopkins RO (2013) Implementation of the pain, agitation, and delirium clinical practice guidelines and promoting patient mobility to prevent post-intensive care syndrome. Crit Care Med 41:S136-45

[21] Suwardianto H (2016) Tardive dyskenesia, motor activity, sedation scale, dan cardiac workload pasien IPI pada pemberian analgesik di instalasi perawatan intensif RS. baptis kediri. Keperawatan Krit. Penelit. Hibah YBI

[22] Morton T (2013) Hyperobjects: Philosophy and Ecology after the End of the World. The Johns Hopkins University Press, USA

[23] Disler RT, White H, Franklin N, Armari E, Jackson D (2019) Reframing evidence-based practice curricula to facilitate engagement in nursing students. Nurse Educ Pract 41:102650

[24] Nathan E B, TD G, Ely, et al (2014) Feasibility and safety of early combined cognitive and physical therapy for critically ill medical and surgical patients: the activity and cognitive therapy in ICU (ACT-ICU) trial. Intensive Care Med 40:370-379

[25] Abelha FJ, Santos CC, Maia PC, Castro MA, Barros H (2007) Quality of life after stay in surgical intensive care unit. BMC Anesthesiol 7:1-12

[26] Bonita A G (2009) Home cardiac rehabilitation for congestive heart failure: a nursing case management approach. Rehabil Nurs 24:143-147

[27] Strahan EH., Brown RJ (2005) A quantitative study of the experiences of patients following transfer from intensive care. Intensive Crit Nursing-ICCN 21:160-171

[28] Ernst, Edzard, Max H. Pittler, Clare Stevinson and AW (2001) The desktop guide to complementary and alternative medicine: an evidence-based approach. White eds London UK 1:459

[29] Nathan E, Brummel, James C. Jackson TDG (2013) A combined early cognititive and physical rehabilitation program for people who are critically Iil: The activity and cognitive therapy in the intensive care unit (ACT-ICU) trial. Phys Ther Crit Illn 92:1580-1592

[30] Suwardianto H, Rimawati (2018) Explicit Instruction Model (EIM): Daily Training Emergencies Preparedness (DTEP) Toward Skills of Participants the Youth Red Cross. Conf 2nd Jt Int 2:403-410

[31] Suwardianto H (2013) Deep breathing relaxation as therapy to decrease blood preassure on hypertension patients. Proc Fac Nurs Airlangga fourd Int Nurs Conf Improv Qual Nurs Care Though Nurs Res Innov 1:1-12

[32] Elliott D, Davidson JE, Harvey MA, et al (2014) Exploring the scope of post–intensive care syndrome therapy and care and Care: engagement of non–critical care Providers and survivors in a second stakeholders meeting. Crit Care Med 42:2518-2526

[33] Christensen H, Batterham PJ, Mackinnon AJ, Jorm AF, Mack HA, Mather KA, Anstey KJ, Sachdev PS, Easteal S (2008) The association of APOE genotype and cognitive decline in interaction with risk factors in a 65-69 year old community

sample. BMC Geriatr. https://doi.org/10.1186/1471-2318-8-14

[34] Kurlowics L, Wallace M (1999) The mini mental state examination (MMSE). Hartford Institude Geriatr Nurs 1:1

[35] Corner EJ, Brett S (2014) Early identification of patien at risk of long-term critical-associatted disability: is it possible? Crit Care 18:629

[36] Lusardi M, Pellecchia G, Schulman M (2003) Functional Performance in Community Living Older Adults. Funct Perform Community Living Older Adults 26:14-22

[37] Society AT (2002) ATS Statement: Guidelines for the Six A Minute Walk Test. Am J Respir Crit Med 166:111-117

[38] Parry SM, Denehy L, Beach LJ, Berney S, Williamson HC, Granger CL (2015) Functional outcomes in ICU – what should we be using? - an observational study. Crit Care. https://doi.org/10.1186/s13054-015-0829-5

[39] Skinner EH, Berney S, Warrilow S, Denehy L (2009) Development of a physical function outcame measure (PFIT) and a pilot exercise training protocol for use in intensive care. Crit Care Resusc 11:110-115

[40] Denehy L, Morton NA de, Skinner EH, Edbrooke L, Haines K, Warrilow S, Berney S (2013) A physical function test for use in the intensive care unit: validity, responsiveness, and predictive utility of the physical function ICU test (scored). Phys Ther 93:1636-1645

[41] Hoppkins R, RR M, L R, Spuhler V, G.E T (2012) Physical therapy on the wards after early physical activity and mobility in the intensive care unit. Phys Ther 92:1518-1523

[42] Bulechek GM, Butcher HK, Dochterman JM, Wagner CM (2013) Nursing interventions classification (NIC), 6th ed. Elsevier Inc, United Kingdom

[43] Smith A, Carey C, Sadler J, Smith H, Stephens R, Frith C (2019) Undergraduate education in anaesthesia, intensive care, pain, and perioperative medicine: The development of a national curriculum framework. Med Teach 41:340-346

[44] Smith MJ, Liehr PR (2014) Middle range theory for nursing thrid edition, 3rd ed. Springer Publishing Company, New York

[45] Suwardianto H, Sari D (2020) Environmental Factors of Sleep Hygiene That Influence The Level of Pain on Criticall ill Patients in Intensive Care Unit. Str J Ilm Kesehat. https://doi.org/10.30994/sjik.v9i1.266

[46] Suwardianto H (2018) Cognitive therapy dengan pendekatan symptom management theory di intensive care unit rs. Baptis kediri. J. Penelit. Keperawatan 4:

[47] Suwardianto H, YC A (2016) Kemandirian Fungsional Lansia Diabetes Melitus Di Kelurahan Bangsal Kota Kediri. J. STIKES RS Baptis Kediri 9:

[48] Suwardianto H, Prasetyo A, Utami RS (2018) Effects of Physical-Cognitive Therapy (PCT) on Criticaly ill Patients in Intensive Care Uni. Hiroshima J Med Sci 67:63-69

[49] Rimawati, Suwardianto H, VW A (2018) Resilience of Knowledge and Perception Skills on the First Aid on Employees. 2nd Jt Int Conf 2:535

[50] Suwardianto H, Sari DAKW (2019) Pain Level in Critical Patients With Sleep Hygiene Care In Intensive Care Unit. J Nurs Pract. https://doi.org/10.30994/jnp.v3i1.61

[51] Suwardianto H (2018) Level Of Perception Emergency Skills In Youth Red Cross. J Nurs Pract 2:17-24

[52] Suwardianto H, Prasetyo A, Utami RS (2017) PHISICAL FUNCTION (MOTOR ACTIVITY) PADA PASIEN KRITIS DENGAN SEDATION DI INTENSIVE CARE UNIT (HASIL TURNITIN).

[53] Suwardianto H Sleep Hygiene, Strategi Mengurangi Tingkat Nyeri Pasien Kritis. Lembaga Chakra Brahmana Lentera

[54] Suwardianto H, Prasetyo A, Utami RS (2017) PHYSICAL COGNITIVE THERAPY MENINGKATKAN FUNGSI FISIK DAN FUNGSI KOGNITIF PASIEN KRITIS DI ICU.

[55] Suwardianto H, Prasetyo A, Utami RS (2017) Phisical Function (Motor Activity) Pada Pasien Kritis Dengan Sedation Di Intensive Care Unit. J Ilmu Kesehat 5:91-102

[56] Astuti VW, Suwardianto H (2016) PENGETAHUAN GURU TAMAN KANAK-KANAK TENTANG ALAT PERMAINAN EDUKATIF DI TAMAN KANAK-KANAK BAPTIS SETIA BAKTI KEDIRI. J. STIKES RS Baptis Kediri 9:

[57] Thomsen GE, Snow GL, Rodhiquez, Ramona, Hopkins (2008) Patients with respiratory failure increase ambulation after transfer to anintensive care unit where early activity is a priority. Crit Care Med 36:1119-1124

[58] Wreksoatmojo BR (2014) Beberapa kondisi fisik dan penyakit yang merupakan faktor resiko gangguan fungsi kognitif. CDK-212 4:25-32

[59] Wijayanti F (2012) Pengaruh terapi kognitif dan latihan asertif terhadap depresi dan kemampuan menguah persepsi diri caregiver Pasien Jantung di RS Jantung Harapan Kita Jakarta.

[60] Balqis UM, Wati NK (2013) Penurunan fungsi kognitif berhubungan dengan ketidakmandirian lansia di Panti Sosual dalam melakukan aktivitas kehidupan sehari-hari. FIK UI 1:1

Section 2

Consciousness and Neural Connectivity

Chapter 4

Brain Functional Architecture and Human Understanding

Yan M. Yufik

> "**Reagan.** *What need one?*
> **King Lear**. *O, reason not the need: our basest beggars*
> *Are in the poorest thing superfluous:*
> *Allow not nature more than nature needs,*
> *Man's life's as cheap as beast's...*"
> *William Shakespeare. King Lear, Act 1, Scene 4*

Abstract

The opening line in Aristotle's *Metaphysics* asserts that "humans desire to understand", establishing understanding as the defining characteristic of the human mind and human species. What is understanding and what role does it play in cognition, what advantages does it confer, what brain mechanisms are involved? The Webster's Dictionary defines understanding as "apprehending general relations in a multitude of particulars." A proposal discussed in this chapter defines understanding as a form of active inference in self-adaptive systems seeking to expand their inference domains while minimizing metabolic costs incurred in the expansions. Under the same proposal, understanding is viewed as an advanced adaptive mechanism involving self-directed construction of mental models establishing relations between domain entities. Understanding complements learning and serves to overcome the inertia of learned behavior when conditions are unfamiliar or deviate from those experienced in the past. While learning is common across all animals, understanding is unique to the human species. This chapter will unpack these notions, focusing on different facets of understanding. The proposal formulates hypotheses regarding the underlying neuronal mechanisms, attempting to assess their plausibility and reconcile them with the recent ideas and findings concerning brain functional architecture.

Keywords: neuronal mechanisms, consciousness, understanding, brain function, functional architecture, neuronal correlations of understanding

1. Introduction

The concept of 'mental models', i.e. memory constructs acting as "small-scale models of reality" intervening between stimuli and responses was introduced in [1], and subsequently elaborated by multiple authors applying the concept in the context of various disciplines [2–6]. More general, domain-invariant theories conceptualize models as inferential frameworks enabling deductive and other forms of reasoning [7, 8], in particular, reasoning by analogy [9].

The theory of understanding discussed in this chapter (the VAN theory formulated in [10–12]) centers on the notions of self-adaptive processes in virtual associative networks (VAN) and defines understanding as a human-specific form of active inference subsumed under the principles of active inference and variational free energy minimization advanced in [13, 14]. The theory contends that curbing metabolic costs and regulating the dynamics of energy processes in the brain have been critical factors in the evolution of intelligence, culminating in the emergence of mental modeling mechanisms in humans that made possible explosive growth in the variety of activities a person can engage in without exploding either the number of neurons and/or the metabolic costs of neuronal processes necessary for organizing those activities. According to the theory, mental models are simultaneous memory structures imposing tight constraints on their constituent components and thus sharply reducing the number of degrees of freedom available to them. Reduction in the number of degrees of freedom minimizes the amount of processing in performing cognitive tasks, yielding two interrelated benefits: curbing energy demands and giving rise to abilities that define human intelligence and are inherent in the understanding capacity, i.e. prediction, explanation, and planning.

These ideas are explored in the present chapter, heeding the advice attributed to Einstein and suggesting that, when pondering a problem, the bulk of the effort needs to be spent on formulating the problem (as clearly as possible). Due to a confluence of circumstances, cognitive science has been downplaying the role of understanding in cognitive performance. The main thrust in this chapter is to examine and elevate that role. The chapter is organized in fours parts. Section 2 reviews challenges to understanding posed by different tasks, Section 3 starts with an excursion into evolutionary history, focusing on differences in cognitive performance making human intelligence discontinuous with that of the other species, and Section 4 outlines a theory of understanding, building on the notions introduced in the preceding parts. Section 5 presents a discussion and brief concluding remarks.

2. Anatomy of understanding

Understanding involves grasping relations between entities, which boils down to fitting representations of these entities into simultaneous memory structures (mental models) that sharply reduce the number of degrees of freedom available to them. Illustrating how these processes operate in the understanding of literary works will help clarifying the ideas.

2.1 Understanding Shakespeare

The corpus of literary work by William Shakespeare includes 37 plays and over 150 sonnets and poems. It has been estimated that a legion of monkeys with as many members as there are protons in the observable universe, each monkey having a typewriter and hitting randomly at the keys, would need the amount of time more than three hundred and sixty thousand orders of magnitude longer than the age of the universe in order to have a negligibly small chance (1 in 10^{500}) of having typed a single play (https://en.wikipedia.org/wiki/Infinite_monkey_theorem).

The adult human brain comprises 86 billion neurons and 85 billion non-neuronal cells [15] which are vanishingly small numbers compared to the size of the monkey legion. How is it possible that a vanishingly small number of cells in Shakespeare's brain managed to produce his entire literary output within a vanishingly small time period (compared to the age of the universe)? The monkey legion is utterly disorganized while the activity of brain cells is precisely orchestrated, what are the principles and mechanisms of such orchestration responsible for the staggering difference in the output? Taking a closer look at the construction of Shakespeare's texts might offer some clues about the organization of brain processes.

Shakespeare's complete works comprise 884,647 words arranged in 118, 406 lines. Applying statistical measures, one can find out, for example, that predictability of letters (entropy per letter) in Shakespeare's texts depends strongly on the letter's position in the word, declining from roughly 3.8 bits in the first letter to 2 bits in the second letter and reaching a plateau of 0.7 bits after the fifth letter. These statistical characteristics are not particularly informative since they do not change much when the words are randomly scrambled, nor there is much difference between Shakespeare's text and a collection of mixed English texts from newspapers [16]. More sophisticated methods of text analysis apply measures of information-based energy and (information-based) temperature to detect variations in the text organization (words with different occurrence frequencies are placed at different energy levels presumed to obey Boltzmann distribution, and the relative temperature of a selected piece of text is computed as the ratio of energy measures in that piece and in the entire corpus). When applied to the collection of Shakespeare's plays, the method revealed that, among the four genres (histories, comedies, tragedies and romances), tragedies have the highest relative temperature (histories have the lowest) and *The Tragedy of Macbeth* scores the highest among the tragedies [17]. How so?

Study in [17] interprets relative temperature as a characteristic of the author's ability to choose words and construct texts in a manner that is both succinct and gives the fullest possible expression to the underlying thoughts (manifesting most prominently in *Macbeth)*. Presumably, exercising this ability in the production of literary works (e.g., writing plays) is aimed at maximizing understandability, that is, affording readers the best means for understanding the author's thoughts and intentions. Understandability can serve as a decisive criteria in assessing differences between Shakespeare's texts and monkeys' output: the overwhelming bulk of monkeys' production is gibberish while Shakespeare's works are understandable and profoundly meaningful.

Per Webster's definition, text understandability depends on the extent to which the selection and composition of words are conducive to a) expressing relations considered by the author and b) constructing relations in the reader's mind isomorphic to those entertained by the author. What is unique about *Macbeth* that could both make the play particularly understandable and also account for the results of statistical analysis? Consider three lines at the apex of the play (scene 23):

> **Seyton.** *The queen, my lord, is dead.*
> **Macbeth.** *She should have died hereafter,*
> *There would have been time for such a word...*

The last two lines present the entirety of Macbeth's reference to the queen in his response to the tragic news; made on the eve of the decisive battle, they convey, in the most succinct and powerful manner, the feeling of despair and a foreboding of the forthcoming military defeat. By wishing to shift the sad news to the "hereafter", Macbeth assigns it a level of significance no lesser than that of the expected military rout and his own likely demise, thus conveying the feeling of a total catastrophe without making any verbose statements to that effect. The following observation concerns a feature of understanding capacity that is presumed to manifest prominently in the cited text, and will play a pivotal role in the theory of understanding outlined in the subsequent sections. Observe that, when constructing the plot, Shakespeare was free to invoke the queens' departure at any point, including allowing her to outlive her husband. The exact timing, neither a day earlier nor at any time "hereafter", must have been decided from the start precisely to motivate the striking expression of despair and the subsequent monolog which expanded the meaning of the play from a chronicle of particular (imaginary) events to a philosophical generalization concerning the inescapable drama of the human condition. The monolog starts with the two lines above and concludes with some of the most quoted passages in Shakespeare's literary legacy.

> *"Life's but a walking shadow; a poor player*
> *That struts and frets his hour upon the stage,*
> *And then is heard no more: it is a tale*
> *Told by an idiot, full of sound and fury,*
> *Signifying nothing."*

The *Tragedy of Macbeth* involves 31 personages, including witches and apparitions, acting in small groupings in 25 consecutive scenes, as shown in **Figure 1**. The sparse matrix in **Figure 1** reveals the overall organization of the play emanating from the organization of the author's mental model that, presumably, formed at the conception of the play and controlled its unfolding.

To underscore, **Figure 1** connotes that, in the mental model, interactions between personages are neither serial nor parallel but simultaneous (or "co-instantaneously co-ordinated", as termed by Jean Piaget in [18]). For example, in scene 3, witches prophesize to Macbeth which results in changing the state of his mind; in scene 7, Macbeth influenced by the prophecy kills Duncan, which was made possible by Duncan's arrival in Macbeth's castle in scene 6, etc. Macbeth's monolog expresses Shakespeare's pessimistic worldview that is echoed in his other plays, for example:

> **Prospero.** *"...Yea, all which is inherit, shall dissolve,*
> *And like this unsubstantial pageant faded,*
> *Leave not a rack behind, we are such stuff*
> *As dreams are made of, and our little life*
> *Is rounded with a sleep." The Tempest, Act 4, scene 1*

Arguably, the corpus of Shakespeare's work, i.e. all 884,647 words in 118, 406 lines, is a congruent expression of a worldview rendering all human affairs, excepting those serving the basic survival needs, both superfluous (see the epigraph to this chapter) and devoid of significance. It appears that exceptionally tight action coordination in the plot of *Macbeth* combined with succinct expressions of the

	Scene 1	....	Scene 3	......	Scene 24	Scene 25
1. Macbeth			1		1	1
2. Lady Macbeth						
3. Macduff					1	
4. Duncan						
5. Malcolm						1
....						
29. First Witch	1		1			
30. Second Witch	1		1			
31. Third Witch	1		1			

Figure 1.
Macbeth *plot comprises tightly coordinated interactions among numerous personages and unfolds in consecutive scenes each involving a subset of personages.*

author's worldview consistent with other such expressions throughout the corpus have surfaced in the text features detected by statistical measures [17].

To summarize what has been suggested up to this point: "apprehending general relations in a multitude of particulars" (per the definition in Webster's Dictionary) takes the form of constructing simultaneous memory structures where entities and their behavior are tightly coordinated. "Relations" are different forms of behavior coordination, i.e., a particular manner in which changes in one entity entail changes in other entities. When entities admit multiple states and a variety of state transitions, relations determine particular mappings between state transition sequences (state trajectories), as shown in **Figure 2**.

Models can form hierarchies where relations in the upper-level models (general relations) admit different instantiations in the lower levels (e.g., a worldview instantiated in different plays). Mental modeling enables predictions, explanations and planning under unfamiliar conditions, by 'running' models to generate predictions and then using predictions to inform the responses. These functions are made possible by coordinations preventing combinatorial explosion that would have made them intractable. One more literary example (adopted from [19]) will help illustrating these important notions.

Two elderly gentlemen, A and B, are waiting together for a train when a presentable looking young man (C) approaches A, politely asking for the time. After a short glance at C, A curtly tells C to leave them alone. When confronted by B about the rude response, A explains: "I thought that if I answered this young man, he might stay with us and keep the conversation going – next, he might board the train with us - next, he might get off the train with us – next, it might happen that my daughter D will come to meet me at the station – next, my daughter and the young man might like each other – next, they might start dating and will eventually marry – next, my daughter might end up unhappy because she married a man who can't even buy himself a watch."

Note that the model was a) composed on the spot to account for a peculiar set of circumstances (as opposed to being retrieved by matching or forged by filling slots in some pre-fabricated template), b) included a chain of tightly coordinated components connecting current conditions to their likely remote consequences (the prediction) and c) enabled using predictions to form a response deviating sharply from the habitual pattern (i.e., rude response to a polite question). More precisely, the model formed by A is a composition of globally coordinated and tightly constrained activities (e.g., C could choose any spot on the platform but was pinned down to the vicinity of A and B, he could board any train and get off anywhere but was constrained to follow A and B, daughter D could be doing anything anywhere but was constrained to appear at the railway station at the time of train's arrival, etc.). The model instantiates a general relation (between income and matrimonial success) held by A, enabling him to predict events in the distant future (D will be unhappy) based on the current cue (C has no watch), and then to use this prediction to inform the immediate response and to explain the prediction and the response to B.

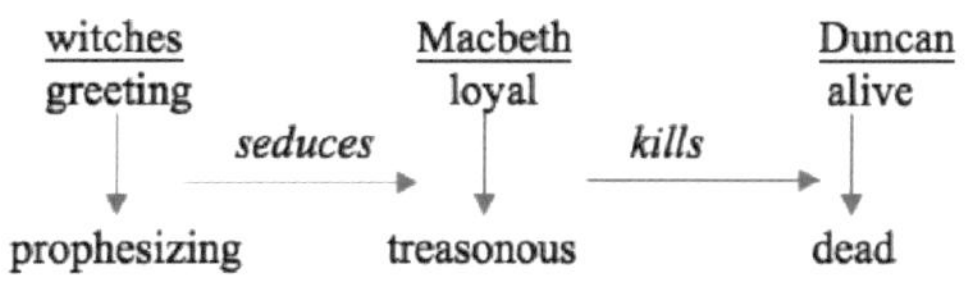

Figure 2.
Relations establish coordinations between state trajectories. Models are simultaneous structures coordinating deployment of relations and self-initiated state changes (e.g., deploying relation "Macbeth kills *Duncan" is preceded by Duncan's decision to put himself in the harm's way, by visiting Macbeth's castle).*

Importantly, models admit deliberately inserted counterfactual variations (e.g. A could have second thoughts and imagine C owning an expensive watch and asking for time because it had accidentally stopped) and generate the corresponding predictions (e.g., a satisfactory marriage) without revisiting the path (i.e., skipping over the sequence "C will stay with us, board the train with us, etc.)). Similarly, the model allows assessing global impact of local changes in one of the components without giving consideration to other components (e.g., one does need to trace the chain of coordinations in order to realize that failure in one element (e.g., D does not come to the station) will fail the entire chain and cancel the prediction). Crucially, models 'resist' relaxation of constraints, requiring forceful (deliberate) insertion of variations (i.e., under the model, the thoughts of D failing to appear, or C owning an expensive watch, etc. do not come to mind, as opposed to being rejected upon examination).

To summarize, eliminating degrees of freedom in mental models entails removing from consideration an otherwise exploding multitude of alternatives, thus making predictions both attainable and usable (i.e., delivered within the time window demanded by the situation). Models admit local variations consistent across the model (e.g. Macbeth's decision to kill Duncan in scene 7 is consistent with what happened to him in scene 2, etc.) and suppress spurious variations. As a result, understanding yields the experience of having succeeded in grasping "general relations in multitudes of particulars", thus turning an intractable mess into a well ordered structure.

The next section turns from literary scenarios to realistic ones, seeking to illustrate the extremes (amazing successes and baffling failures) in the operation of understanding.

2.2 From children's games to revolutionary discoveries

2.2.1 Baffling failures

Children at an early age often fail to connect and coordinate events taking place right in front of them, as follows. The child is shown a toy which is subsequently placed under a cover allowing her to retrieve the toy. After a few successful repetitions, the toy is transferred, in full view of the child, to another spot where it is placed under another cover. After some hesitation, the child looks for the toy, not in the spot to where it was just moved but in the previous one [20].

Claudius Galen, an outstanding philosopher and physician in the Roman Empire, formulated a theory of blood production and processing in the body (circa 150 AD). The theory asserted that blood is produced in the liver from ingested food, rises to the lungs through the right side of the heart, crosses through pores to the left side where it is mixed with inhaled air and, finally, gets distributed throughout the body and consumed by the tissue (the surplus is expelled with sweat and urine). In this schema, heart remains a reservoir where blood is collected and treated (mixed with air) on its way from the source (liver) to the sink (tissues). In the XIth century, Galen's works were translated into Latin and became a dogma that dominated medical profession for over 500 years. Ironically, bloodletting was one of the most frequent treatment modalities in the medieval medicine, but neither the viewing of blood streams spurting from incisions nor the evidence of heart's incessant beating in one's own chest could cause questioning of the dogma. In 1628, English physician William Harvey published a book presenting a simple and cogently argued model of blood circulation. Moreover, he pointed out absurdities inherent in the dogma (e.g., the liver would have to produce several times the body weight in blood every day if the blood was being absorbed). Despite their undeniable strength (a simple model accounting fully of the available data and revealing critical shortcomings in the earlier account), Harvey's ideas were met with ridicule [21, 22]. The medical profession was unable to overcome the inertia and re-structure the entrenched model, thus failing to apprehend coordination between a few vital variables. Galen was an expert on pulse diagnosis and published a treaties on the subject, which makes his conceptual blind spots particularly baffling. Perpetuation of Galen's model would have arrested progress in medicine, causing incalculable losses (think of Galenic cardiology).

2.2.2 Spectacular successes

In the 1820–1835 time period, Michael Faraday formulated key ideas of the field theory postulating relations between electric and magnetic phenomena which, in the preceding decades, were commonly viewed as being totally unrelated. Expressed in a mathematical formalism by James Clerk Maxwell, the Faraday - Maxwell model of electromagnetism depicted propagation of electric and magnetic fields as tightly coordinated processes. Faraday's conceptualization of fields envisioned material entities of a kind that are not perceptually accessible but permeate space and carry force. In a brilliant feat of expansive insight, Maxwell realized the existence of relations between electromagnetic waves, light and perception of color. These findings have been propelling advances in physics and technology, until the present day and into the foreseeable future.

Modern physics (quantum mechanics, astrophysics) deals with entities that are not directly observable. Literature reports that key ideas concerning quantum processes were formulated by Werner Heisenberg (circa 1925) following an insight he allegedly received when taking a walk in the park at night and observing a passer by appearing in illuminated areas under lamp posts and disappearing in the shadows when leaving those areas [23]. The position and movement of the person between the posts remained undetermined, suggesting the idea of indeterminate states of electrons in the atom when transiting between energy levels (somewhat similar to indeterminate states of characters in a play when transiting between scenes, as in **Figure 1**). Quantum mechanics proved to be the most successful physical theory ever formulated, predicting the outcomes of particle interactions with unparalleled accuracy.

As reported in [24], an explosion on a DC-10 passenger airliner incapacitated one of three engines and demolished the hydraulic system, causing loss of control mechanisms for the remaining two engines except for their thrust levers. Hydraulic systems are built with triple redundancy, bringing the odds of losing control due to hydraulic system failure to less than one in a billion. Accordingly, no protocol has been ever created for handling such occasions and no training was ever offered. When the aircraft started pitching violently up and down (a phugoid pattern), the pilot had a short time window to figure out how to suppress phugoids and land the aircraft. According to pilot's recollections, a simplified model was formed in his mind that accounted for the location of the remaining two engines and suggested a maneuvering strategy using differential thrust. The strategy was not only unfamiliar but grossly counterintuitive, requiring decelerating when the aircraft was climbing and accelerating when it was heading down. When flight conditions were reproduced in a simulator, numerous pilots failed to figuring out a course of action and kept crashing (could not make the runway after dozens of attempts) [24].

Samuel Reschevsky, a chess prodigy born in 1911 in Poland, learned the game at the age of four and at the age of eight was defeating champions of his country in tournaments, as well as beating scores of opponents, including master-level players, in public demonstrations of simultaneous play. Although cognitive difficulties faced in chess have been always appreciated, there were no satisfactory methods for quantifying them until the era of chess computers. Chess algorithms required hardware with operating speed at or above 10^8 position evaluations per second in order to compete with expert players capable of carrying out at most one or two position evaluations per second. Understanding the game compensates for the 1: 10^8 disadvantage in speed: expert players perceive configurations of pieces as compositions of "complexes", deriving game plans from apprehending coordinations between the "complexes" [25]. Findings in [25] suggest that expert game models take the form of simultaneous structures, not unlike the matrix in **Figure 1**. A novice's perception is limited to a few adjacent cells in the matrix (2–3 moves look-ahead involving 2–3 pieces) while expert models can include a hierarchy of matrices encompassing the entire configuration and extending to 10–15 moves look-ahead Position analysis involves envisioning variations for some of the moves, constrained by the entire web of coordinations across the matrix. As a result, experts are not distracted into considering spurious (weak) moves, no more than novices waste effort in considering illegal moves [26].

To summarize, the previous section associated understanding with the development of mental models representing entities, their behavior and different forms of behavior coordination in the form of simultaneous memory structures. It was suggested that simultaneous coordination suppresses combinatorial explosion, confining the process to an infinitesimally small volume in the vast combinatorial space (considering possible move combinations in chess, similar to considering possible letter combinations in playwriting, quickly brings one to the realm of counting protons in multiple universes). Prediction, explanation and planning are enabled by mental modeling. This section reviewed extreme cases when modeling processes failed to establish coordination between a few directly observable and persistent entities and succeeded in quickly coordinating multiple, transient and/or unobservable ones. Summarily, suggestions and observations in Section 2 define the main challenges facing a theory of understanding:

a. what neuronal mechanisms can account for the successes and shortcomings of the understanding capacity,

b. how such mechanisms could emerge and

c. how could they develop in the human species within the time period of negligible duration (on the evolutionary time scale).

The next part focuses on the emergence of understanding.

3. A brief history of understanding

Notions addressed in this part were developed elsewhere [10–13, 27–30] and will be summarized briefly here. A preview will help putting the notions together: Environment is in flux, survival depends on an organism's ability to adapt to the changing environment. Adaptation makes the world livable while understanding makes it intelligible, that is, amenable to prediction and explanation (i.e., connecting likely future events to their plausible causes in the past and present). Mechanisms of understanding complete the transformation of sensory streams into world models that generate such predictions and explanations. The transformation starts with mechanisms of sensation and perception that are available, in different forms, in other species, and culminates in the mechanism of understanding unique to humans. Learning response-reward (response-punishment) patterns increases reward chances and decreases punishment risks when conditions recur. A repertoire of such learned patterns constitutes a model of the environment instantiated by pattern matching. Understanding is an advanced adaptive mechanism serving to overcome the inertia of prior learning and optimize responses when conditions are novel or violate the previously acquired conditions-response associations in a consequential manner (e.g., learned responses cease to be rewarding) [10–13]. This characterization is consistent with definitions of intelligence in the literature ("fluid intelligence" [18, 31–33]) establishing understanding capacity as the central, defining feature of human intellect.

3.1 Evolutionary precursors

Complex life forms have been developing on Earth at an accelerating pace: From the emergence of unicellular organisms some 3.7 billion years ago, to (the emergence of) multicellular animals 900 million years ago, to vertebrate 530 million years ago, to primates about 70 million years ago, to the detachment of the human branch from the chimpanzee/bonobos primate branch 6 million years ago to, finally, the emergence of anatomically modern Sapiens [34] at the time period of 200,000–100,000 years ago (the emergence of language is attributed to the time period of roughly 150,000–60,000 years ago [35–37].

Recent findings indicated genealogical continuity in Sapience in the last 28,000 years, i.e. from Upper Paleolithic to modern times [38]. During the same period, the size of the braincase has been decreasing, having lost more than 10% of its peak value [39]), after a preceding period of about 6 million years during which the size almost tripled [40]. Recent analysis comparing the results of electrophysiological, anatomical and fMRI studies in humans and non-human primates associated development of intelligence primarily with reorganization of brain mechanisms [41]. These findings seem to indicate that reorganizations entailed higher efficiency so that progressively more complex tasks could be carried out

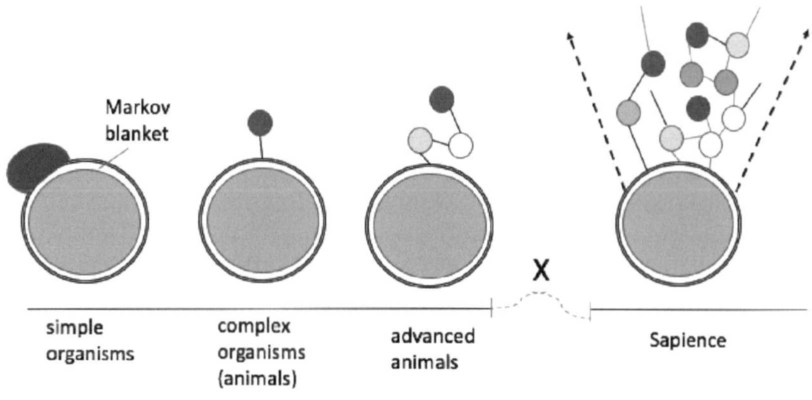

Figure 3.
Gap X denotes discontinuity in the development of cognitive capacities. Simple organisms interact with substances located on their 'blankets', more complex organisms can move towards and reach for target objects (denoted by black circles) in close proximity to their blankets (e.g. salamanders shoot their tongues to catch insects), and advanced animals (apes, some avians) can use a few supplementary objects (denoted by shaded and white circles) to act on the target (e.g. chimpanzees can connect sticks and pile up boxes in order to reach a hanging fruit). Humans are discontinuous with the other species in that they can form coordinated structures (designs) comprising indefinitely large sets of supplementary objects giving access to indefinitely distant targets, with the possibility of postponing acting on such targets until some indefinitely remote future moments (anticipatory planning).

without increasing the size of the neuronal pool. Section 4 will suggest the type of reorganization that could produce such revolutionary improvements.

Comparing modes of interaction between the organism and environment across the spectrum of life forms reveals discontinuities between Sapiens and other species, as shown in **Figure 3**. The term 'Markov blanket' [13, 14] denotes an enclosing boundary (e.g., membrane) separating organism from the environment (the notion will be defined more precisely in the next section).

Differences between Sapience and other species are qualitative: they lie not in the increased quantity of supplementary objects but in the drive to keep extending the reach of action (action envelope) and to form progressively more complex designs comprising growing numbers of objects of increasing variety. Stated differently, animal envelopes are limited to the immediate proximity of their Markov blankets while human envelopes undergo indefinite expansion. Amplifying Shakespeare's insight (expressed succinctly in the epigraph), it can be suggested that animals seek biological equilibrium with their environment (i.e., maintaining inflows of energy and nutrients at life-sustaining levels) while humans seek cognitive equilibrium entailing demands not reducible to those associated with sustaining life. Hence, gap X. What is the nature of that gap?

3.1.1 Learning and pattern recognition

Consider challenges facing organisms in a changing environment. Assume first that the varying flow of conditions (stimuli) includes some recurring patterns. Since finding successful responses consumes time and effort, recognizing such patterns and re-using the responses saves both. The strategy works best when patterns comprise a few contiguous stimuli that trigger a small repertoire of fixed responses. However, even this simple strategy working under favorable circumstances can become self-defeating when the circumstance change, as illustrated in the following example.

Salamanders shoot their tongues at objects (insects) whose size, speed and distance from the animal fall within some fixed ranges, which requires anticipatory response control (early activation of the projector muscle relative to the tongue launch) to improve the chances of successful intercepts. The shooting mechanism was fine-tuned by evolution (developing spring-loaded type of tongue ejection yielding high energy output), making the animal a successful predator [42]. Consider a hypothetical scenario when the advantages are turned into detriments. The shooting mechanism is thermally sensitive: the speed of tongue retraction increases with temperature [42] which can be used, potentially, to increase the amount of prey intake per unit time. Assume that the animal can learn the 'higher temperature – higher intake' association, compelling it to seek high temperature spots. Such learning will keep paying off for as long as the prey cooperates: if the insects start moving faster in the vicinity of hot spots (or avoid them, etc.), the intercept success rate will decline. However, the animal will be bound to continue the heat-seeking behavior until the association decays, which might cause it to die from hunger and/or exhaustion (missing targets decreases food intake but not the costs). The point is that the ability to suppress learned behavior can yield quantum leap improvements in adaptive robustness, by reducing the probability of 'blind persistence' types of error inherent in recognition-centered strategy, and/or reducing the severity of the consequences. In general, the strategy works if short contiguous patterns (compact patterns) recur with frequency sufficient for satisfying the organism's survival needs. Assume that the requirement is not met, forcing the animal to seek strategies applicable in more complex stimuli configurations.

3.1.2 Gap X

Removing (or relaxing) the contiguity requirement changes an animal's view of the environment: form a noisy stream of compact patterns to a stream of uncertain structure where patterns can no longer be readily discerned. Stated differently, in streams of non-contiguous patterns (dispersed patterns) stimuli groupings in one pattern can be interspersed irregularly with groupings belonging to other patterns, thus allowing extending patterns over indefinitely long stimuli sequences and time periods. Dispersed patterns place organisms at the horns of a dilemma, as shown below.

Pattern composition in **Figure 4(2)** is inherently uncertain, gradual reduction of the uncertainty proceeds reversibly through the stages of a) defining entities (as compositions of states), b) defining behaviors (as patterns of state transition) c) defining relations (as forms of behavior coordination), resulting in the construction of simultaneous structures representing interactions between entities in successions of episodes, as shown in **Figure 5**.

Strategies in **Figure 4(1)** and **(2)** reside at the opposite sides of gap X: cognitive operations underlying the former are exogenously driven, i.e., triggered by the environment and carried out under feedback control, while operations underlying the latter are endogenously-driven, i.e. decoupled from the sensory inflows. Rudimentary forms of such decoupling manifest in animal behavior, e.g., dogs following a prey that disappears behind an obstacle might not chase it around the corner but run to intercept at the opposite corner. On the human side of the gap, reversible operations become available gradually as the person matures, causing characteristic errors (e.g., young children fail in the "toy has moved" task requiring that association (toy, cover1, spot1) is followed by dissociation (toy, cover1, spot1) ➔ (cover 1, spot 1) ➔ (toy, cover2, spot2), see section I.2.a. A different form of dissociation deficit manifests in older children when they fail to dissociate container from the contents: a child watching liquid being poured from one container to another can believe that the amount changes with the size of the container [43].

Note that entity construction principles in **Figure 4(2)** and **5** express an implicit assumption that entity's identity can be preserved in different manifestations in non-contiguous episodes, that is, the same entity can have different (non-overlapping) manifestations and, vice versa, different entities can have identical manifestations (e.g., in Greek mythology, enterprising Zeus was appearing to mortal women in the form of a swan, a bull, or even a shower. On one occasion, Zeus presented himself to a lady in a form that was identical to her husband (Amphitryon) in every

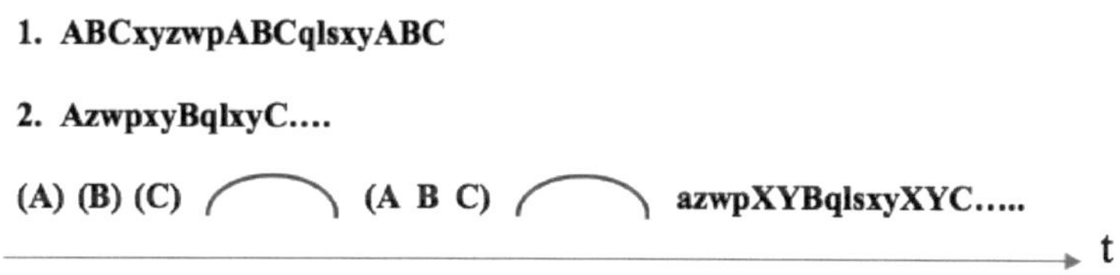

Figure 4.
Transition from compact to dispersed patterns inside gap X. 1) contiguous stimuli grouping ABC recurs at irregular noisy intervals, response strategy consists in finding activities rewarded by ABC and emitting them whenever the pattern is recognized. 2) removing the contiguity requirement changes the strategy from pattern recognition to pattern construction. Here is the dilemma: stimuli A, B, C can be manifestations of either different entities requiring different responses **or** *different states of the same entity requiring the same response (possibly, with modifications). Whatever the resolution, it might change at some later point in time, e.g. XYB and XYC can be determined to be the states of some entity Z, causing a to recede into the background noise, etc.*

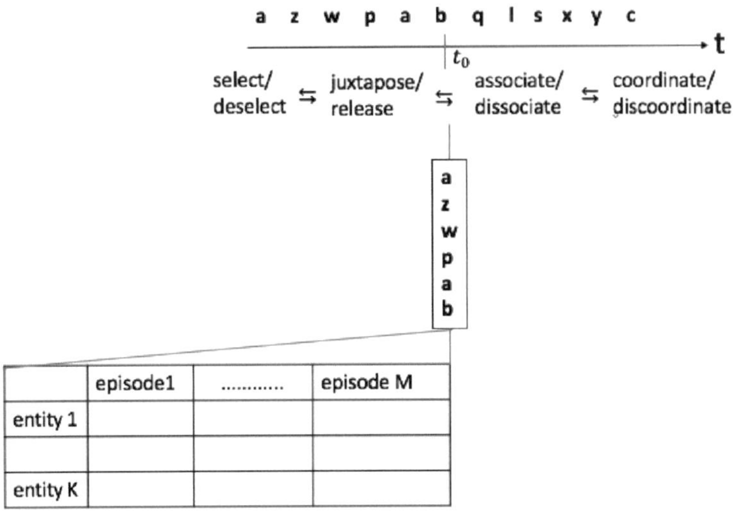

Figure 5.
An irreversible stimuli stream is transformed into a simultaneous record, cycles of reversible operations on the record (select/deselect, etc.) produce simultaneous structures comprising various entities interacting in series of episodes (see ***Figure 1****).*

detail but was not her husband – Amphitryon was quite sure of that). Implicit explorations of logic in Greek mythology were made explicit by Aristotle in the Laws of Thought, including the Law of Identity.

3.2 Crossing gap X

According to an appealing hypothesis [44], the earliest steps in the expansion of the human envelope were associated with predation by throwing projectiles (stones). Accurate aiming requires precise coordination of several variables including launch angle, velocity, weight and size of the stone, distance to the prey and its size, and release time, with the width of the release time window limited to a few milliseconds (e.g., 11 milliseconds for a rabbit-size stationary target located 4 meters away, these results will be re-visited in the next section). Analysis based on experimental findings (narrowing the time window involves synchronization in neuronal clusters of growing size) demonstrated that increasing distance to targets while maintaining the hit rate requires explosive growth in the number of neurons responsible for precise timing (64-fold and 729-fold increase in the number of neurons to double and triple the distance, correspondingly).

Anatomical limitations imposed on the volume of cranial cavity appeared to exclude the possibility that a growing variety of high-precision activities (e.g. splitting stones for different tasks) could be obtained by developing narrowly specialized neuronal modules. Anatomical limitations enforce other trade-offs having impact on cognitive performance, e.g., increasing the speed of pulse conduction would require increasing the thickness of myelin wrappings, which would decrease the number of neurons the cranial geometry can accommodate [40, 44] .

In addition to constraints in brain size and conduction speed, another physical factor having decisive impact on brain processes is limited supply of energy for powering them. Since physical constraints on brain processes are non-negotiable, the only avenue for obtaining quantum advancements in cognitive performance depicted in **Figure 2** appears to be dynamic optimization in their deployment, which boils down to global coordination via the mechanisms of mental modeling.

DOI: http://dx.doi.org/10.5772/intechopen.95594

These notions will be addressed in the theory of understanding in the next part, following another example of mental modeling in the closing of this part.

For the sake of argument, assume that advancing the predation-by-throwing-projectiles strategy involved invention of catapults, in the simplest form of a board (B1) balanced on a base, or fulcrum (B2). Note that neither component, if considered individually, betrays any hint as to its potential usefulness for projectile throwing. Moreover, when considered jointly, these components afford numerous arrangements that are all useless (e.g., the base on top of the board, etc.), with only one particular form of base-board position coordination yielding the benefit. Operations involved in constructing and operating catapults are suggested in **Figure 6**.

Note that the product of modeling is a new entity (a weapon) that has properties unavailable in the components and expands the activity envelope (larger distances, heavier projectiles). Running the model yields understanding, i.e., informs operation and aiming procedures. For example, envisioning one side of the board going up brings to mind the image of the other side going down, envisioning increasing the distance to the target brings to mind the image of increasing the length of the shoulder (shifting the projectile away from the base), etc. That same process underlies prediction (e.g. hit probability) and explanation (why hitting that target over there is unlikely?).

It is interesting to note that children up to a certain age, when learning to operate toy catapults, are often incapable of forming proper models and keep shifting projectiles in the direction of the target as it moves away (shortening the shoulder), even after having watched the proper operation multiple times [43]. The instinctual tendency to grasp receding objects by extending arms and moving after the objects resists learning. Young children cannot understand catapults.

Recent theories concerning the origins of language placed the capacity to perform reversible juxtaposition (operation Merge) at the foundation on which all other language mechanisms have been built (B2 B1) ➔ C (operation Merge combines syntactic objects in an arbitrary order [45]).

To summarize, this part defined understanding as an advanced adaptive mechanism that makes possible constructing responses to indefinitely large patterns comprised of non-contiguous stimuli groupings (dispersed patterns). Construction proceeds through identifying entities, their properties and behavior and the forms of inter-entity behavior coordination, culminating in the production of simultaneous, tightly coordinated structures comprising multiple entities (mental models). Models are amenable to manipulations, giving rise to the dual capacity for predicting likely events (changes in the entities) and identifying their causes in the past or present (explanations). In general, any organism can be viewed as a cast molded by the environmental niche it occupies, e.g., salamander is a 'cast mold' of environment where particular (edible) insects having size and speed within some fixed ranges are flowing into a volume in space reachable by the animal in unit time in quantities sufficient for the animal's survival. The total model includes biophysical component

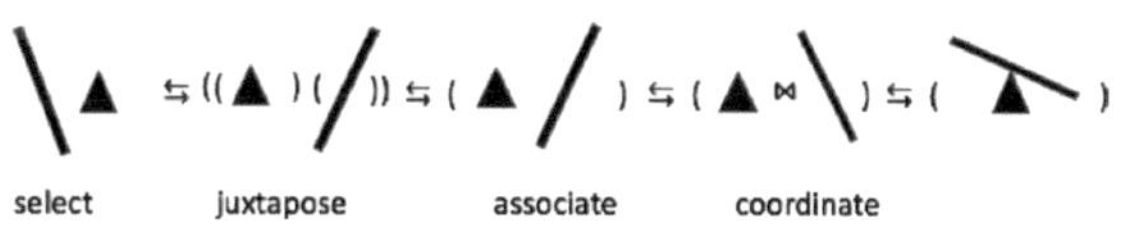

Figure 6.
Modeling starts with selecting entities (objects) and juxtaposing them as separate (independent) entities, followed by associating them in a composite structure allowing inter-dependence, followed by coordinating the entities to form a model (note that juxtaposition brings components together in an arbitrary order while association imposes order, setting the stage for establishing a higher degree of order in the model). Symbol ⋈ denotes coordination.

(body and the sensory-motor periphery, e.g. the tongue-ejecting mechanism) and regulatory component orchestrating activities within the body and at the periphery (i.e., animal's behavior in the environment). Both components undergo evolutionary development in the species while behavior regulation is amenable to adaptive changes in individuals during their lifetime (learning). In animals, learning is restricted to condition-driven variations within narrow envelopes of genetically-fixed condition-response patterns and propensities. Condition-driven learning extrapolates from past precedents while mental modeling enables prediction and response construction under conditions having no such precedents. More precisely, models integrate past history within cross-coordinated structures so predictions produced by operations on the structure can be made consistent with (plausible under the entire past history) without repeating any of its elements. Moreover, models allow reproductive construction without replication, e.g., coordinations in the basic catapult were reproduced in numerous designs.

As observed by Jean Piaget [46].

> *"...mental coordinations succeed in combining all the multifarious data and successive data into an overall, simultaneous picture, which vastly multiplies their powers of spatio-temporal extension, and of deducing possible developments"*
> *([46] p. 218).*

Summarily, it has been suggested that a) the protohuman-to-human transition was associated with the emergent capacity to construct responses to dispersed stimuli patterns and b) the capacity is rooted in the mechanisms of mental modeling that represents such patterns as coordinated structures that suppress combinatorial explosion inherent in the construction process and reduce the number of response compositions to a few plausible alternatives.

4. Theory of understanding: neuronal mechanisms of mental modeling

The theory in a nutshell: Nervous system optimizes deployment of sensory-motor resources vis-à-vis varying external conditions, a part of the system that coordinates variations in the deployment of sensory motor-resources with variations in the conditions flow constitutes the first regulatory loop. Mechanisms of understanding operate on top of the first loop and optimize the organization of neuronal resources engaged in that loop, thus forming the second regulatory loop. Optimization in the second loop involves arranging neurons into coordinated structures manifested in coordinated mental models, as shown in **Figure 4**. Operations in the first loop are controlled by sensory-motor feedback while operations in the second one are decoupled from it. Feedback control makes resource deployment adaptive, self-controlled optimization in the second loop makes it self-adaptive [11]. First and second loops are stages of self-organization in the neuronal substrate. The first loop allows adaptation to compact sensory patterns extending over short time periods while the second one expands adaptation to dispersed patterns extending over indefinitely large time periods (prediction). limitations on the size of the neuronal pool and the amount of usable energy supplied per unit time drive the need to increase adaptation span while reducing energy costs, which boils down to a dual optimization criteria: minimize energy losses and the amount of energy consuming activities while maximizing prediction accuracy. Both criteria are subsumed under the notion of active inference [13, 14, 47].

This part will discuss the role of understanding capacity within the active inference framework, followed by detailed suggestions regarding neuronal mechanisms that underlie the capacity and are responsible for the range of its operation, including the extremes. The part concludes by referencing experimental findings and ideas in the literature that might help in assessing biological plausibility of the present proposal.

4.1 Active inference: from Aristotle to Friston

The opening line in Aristotle's *Metaphysics* states that "humans desire to understand" [48]. Lack of understanding engenders puzzlement, and failure to identify causes leads to undesirable self-evaluation

> *".. men of experience know that thing is so, but do not know why, while the others know the 'why' and the cause.... and man who is puzzled and wonders thinks himself ignorant" (Aristotle, Metaphysics).*

In a penetrating insight, Aristotle captures relations between experiences, surprise (puzzlement) and self-directed activities motivated by the desire to reach beyond the appearances (identify causes). Arguably, principles of active inference and variational free energy minimization advanced in [13] are congruent with those early insights. The principles assert that life in all its forms, from unicellular organisms to humans, is predicated on the organisms ability to use sensing to predict conditions in its environment and to conduct activities reducing the difference between the predicted and the actual experiences. Predictions require models of the environment, the variational free energy value determines, roughly, the (information-theoretic) distance between the current and the desired states that takes into account the difference between the predicted conditions and those that were actually sensed and the surprise experienced under the model (the smaller the probability assigned by the model to the condition, the higher the surprise).

Emphasis on activities directed at minimizing variational free energy underlies the notion of 'active inference,' which is best appreciated if contrasted to the idea of 'passive' inference expressed in Plato's allegory of the cave, as follows. Prisoners are chained to the floor inside a cave where they can see nothing of the outside world except shadows on the wall they are facing. The message is that people are caged inside their minds, senses are the only window into the world, and that window can be distorting. The allegory defines passive inference: prisoners can make guesses about the outside world but have no means to validate them or to use in any fashion.

Active inference differs from passive inference in that it incorporates iterative actions on both the outside world and the model of that world that can lead to progressively improving guesses. Understanding involves a form of model manipulation that is best defined within the active inference theory through the notion of a Markov Blanket - the third conceptual pillar in the theory integrating ideas about emergence of life, evolution, and brain operation into a seamless whole.

'Markov Blanket of node x' is a graph-theoretic term denoting a set of nodes in a directed graph that are connected to x by links incident to and from x. More loosely, the term can be used to denote a group of nodes in subnetwork X1 separating it from the rest of the network X. If links denote some form of interaction, Markov Blanket of X1 can be viewed as an interface through which internal nodes in X1 interact with their surrounds in X. On that view, Markov Blanket accords X1 a degree of (conditional) independence from X - a critical concept in the overall theory, as follows.

The theory of life attributes emergence of life to spontaneous phase transitions in molecular networks ('primordial soup'), resulting in the formation of subnetworks that remain connected to their surrounds but acquire a degree statistical

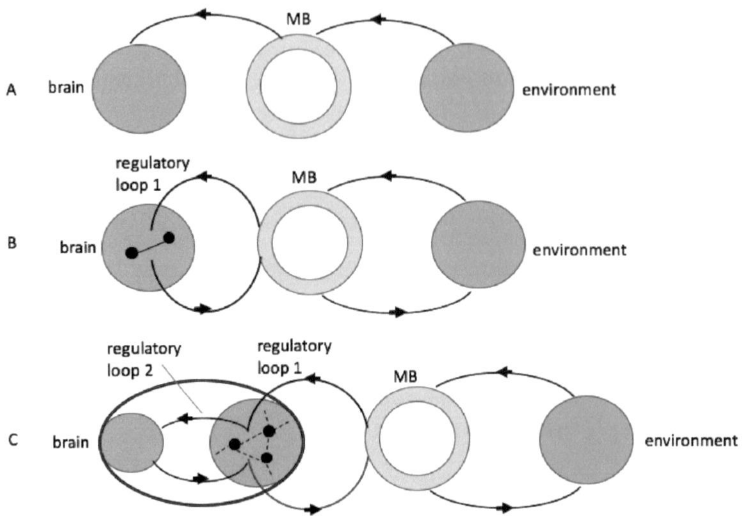

Figure 7.
Passive inference, active inference and comprehensive active inference. (A) The allegory of the cave (passive observation without action: sensory input is neither solicited nor acted upon. (B) Observation-action iterations guided by feedback produce (deposit) a model that adjusts subsequent iterations and gets adjusted by them. (C) Second regulatory loop manipulates structures formed by the first loop to construct models, the process is decoupled from the motor-sensory feedback.

independence (autonomy) from it. In that context, Markov Blanket denotes interface (a 'membrane') between such quasi-autonomous formations and their environment [14]. As more complex forms of life develop, the Markov Blanket expands to incorporate the entire sensory-motor periphery, as suggested in **Figure 3**. Finally, **Figure 7** separates Markov Blanket from the nervous system to illustrate the notions of active inference and comprehensive active inference (incorporating the understanding capacity).

The process in **Figure 7A** is an idealization; **Figure 7B** depicts associative learning (e.g. the hypothetical salamander associates elevated temperature with successful hunting, entailing search for hot spots); **Figure 7C** depicts active construction of mental models that underlies understanding. Learning yields "knowledge that a thing is so", understanding defines causes.

In summary, different facets of the ideas depicted in **Figure 7** have been addressed in numerous sources in psychology, physiology, neuroscience and philosophy of the mind. The active inference framework offers a synthesis of some of the key insights in these disciplines, integrating them in a coordinated conceptual structure expressed in a unifying mathematical formalism. The central notion is that of activity: an organism is actively seeking sensory inputs, constructs models and acts on the environment. These contentions will be re-visited in the discussion.

4.2 Neuronal mechanisms

The proposal in this section stems from five assumptions about the nature of neuronal processes that underlie intelligence and its special form, understanding. The proposal will be presented in three sections: first, the assumptions are formulated, along with some clarifications; next, the key points in the theory are formulated and applied to answer questions posed at the end of Section 2; finally, these key points are re-visited and related to experimental findings and other ideas in the literature.

4.2.1 Assumptions

4.2.1.1 Cognition involves active deployment of neuronal resources

Brain is a synergistic system that selects, mobilizes and deploys (fires) neurons. Mobilization involves activities that precede firing and are centered on tuning, as shown **Figure 8**.

Consider the following three experiments: raising your right hand and touching your nose with the index finger, doing the same with your eyes closed, and imagining the same without doing anything. The first run involves coordination in the external space, the second involves coordination in the mental space (you know where your nose and your finger are, without reference to external coordinates), the third demonstrates coordination in the neuronal space that underlies the other two (I shall return to these exciting experiments at the end of the section).

4.2.1.2 Progressively improving deployment requires relative stability of neuronal groups

Deployment strategy progresses from deploying individual neurons to deploying neuronal groups, to deploying groups of groups, etc., which requires a degree of stability in all the elements of the growing organization. This intuition entailed the notion of "neuronal packets" that is pivotal in the theory.

A neuronal packet is Hebb's assembly (i.e., comprises neurons connected by associative links) that is synergistic and is separated by a boundary energy barrier from the surrounding associative network.

It was hypothesized that packets form as a result of phase transition in associative networks, not unlike raindrops form in vapor. Accordingly, energy barrier is determined by surface tension, that is, the amount of free energy per unit surface (presumably, surface comprises cell membranes in the boundary neurons. Accordingly, surface energy is determined by the distribution of membrane potential across the surface). Neurons at the packet boundary constitute packet's Markov Blanket, surface tension in the boundary holds neurons together. Mapping these notions on the process in **Figure 4** will help appreciating its crucial consequences: first, combining neurons responding to A, B, C, D, E... in a quasi-stable bounded packet amounts to asserting existence (perceiving) some bounded entity (object) α comprising features α = {A, B, C, D, E...} and, second, synergistic packets allow 'tuning' to their

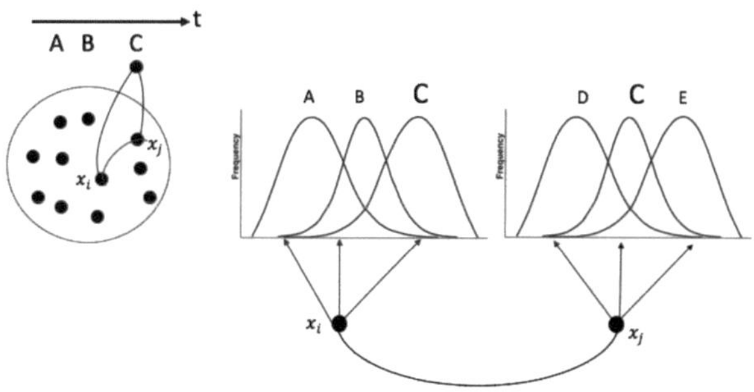

Figure 8.
Neurons x_i and x_j are selected in the neuronal pool and tuned to stimulus C in the stimuli stream. Neuron x_i responds to A, B, C stimuli, tuning amplifies its response to C. Sensing and motor actions are both products of active deployment (e.g. one sees color C because some neurons were selected, mobilized and tuned to C). Imagining color C involves the same process. Imagining A, or B, or C involves shifts in tuning, which can be expressed as rotating neuron's response vector. Co-firing of x_i and x_j establishes an associative link between them.

individual constituents (rotating packet vector) which is experienced as envisioning different states, or facets of object α (e.g., rotating the image). Energy barriers 'anchor' determinations in Figure 4, e.g., once feature A has been attributed to object α , the barriers will resist (require energy investment in) separating A from α . As a result, barriers serve the dual function of binding neurons together in stable groups and binding those groups to 'objects.' **Figure 9** illustrates these notions.

4.2.1.3 Improving deployment requires coordination of neuronal groups

Models are composite 'objects,' i.e., synergistic groups of coordinated packets. For example, neuronal group 'catapult' comprises packets 'board', 'base', 'projectile' and 'target' and can be 'tuned' to different states of the composite object. A crucial point: feature space of 'catapult' has dimensionality higher than that of the constituents, rotating the 'catapult' vector (e. g, switching between states 'unloaded'➔ 'loaded' ➔ 'aimed', etc.) reflects coordinated movement of the constituent vectors (e.g., envisioning a receding target brings to mind the image of a projectile moving away from the base). **Figure 10** maps these notions on the organization depicted in **Figure 7c**.

4.2.1.4 Brain is a self-organizing virtual system

Genetically-defined propensities in the brain substrate (gray and white matter, etc.) allow a range of self-organization trajectories, the actual developmental

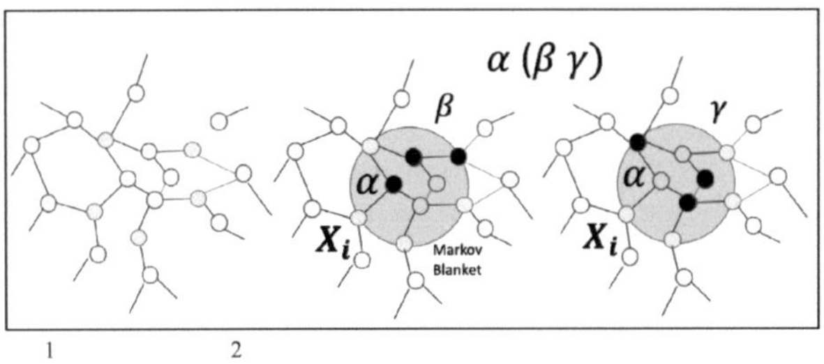

Figure 9.
1. Successive co-activation of different neurons produces a growing associative network. 2. Associative network undergoes phase transition resulting in the formation of packet X_i , giving rise to perceiving object α . Different activation–inhibition patterns in α underlie the experience of α manifesting states β and γ and behavior patterns) β ➔ γ and γ ➔ β .

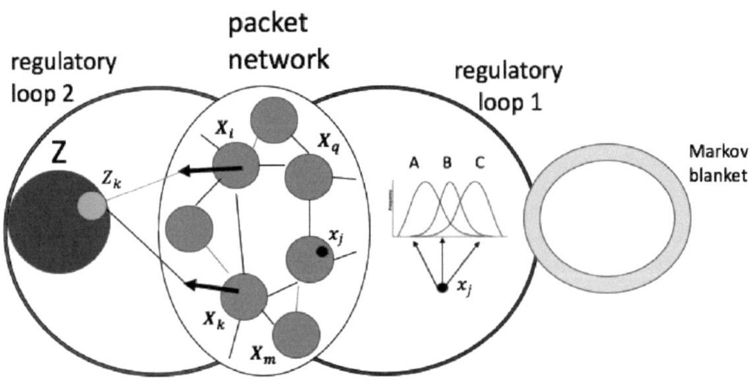

Figure 10.
Phase transitions in the associative network transform it into a packet network. Selecting, mobilizing and deploying packets in the packet network populates the world with a multitude of distinct objects capable of different behavior patterns. Mental models establish coordination between behavior patterns.

trajectory results from an interplay between the propensities and conditions encountered throughout the lifetime.

4.2.1.5 Brain is an energy seeking system

Self-organization is predicated on energy inflows sufficient for producing coordinated neuronal structures. The process is sustainable because it stabilizes energy inflows via expanding the range of extremal activities (thus diversifying energy sources) while minimizing internal energy expenditures incurred in the expansion.

4.2.1.6 Self-organization proceeds through assimilation/accommodation cycles

Periods of deliberate (attentive, self-directed) construction and manipulation of mental models alternate with periods of spontaneous re-structuring: the overall neuronal organization adapts to the newly formed structures and, reciprocally, the new structure are adjusted and integrated into the organization.

4.2.1.7 Brain is a synergistic system

In neuronal structures, a few controls can manipulate a much larger numbers of degrees of freedom [49, 50]. **Figure 11** illustrates this important notion.

4.2.2 Putting it all together: neuronal substrate of understanding and brain functional architecture

Assumptions advanced in the preceding section entail the following suggestions.

1. Formation of neuronal packets transforms associative network into a packet network embedded into an energy landscape, with the packets residing in local minima. The height of packet energy barrier E_m (free energy) is a function of temperature T and parameter $\sigma(T)$ reflecting cumulative strength of associative links incident to the packet's Markov Blanket (MB) from inside the packet vs. the cumulative strength of those incident from the outside.

$$E_m = \sigma(T) - T\, d\sigma(T) / dT$$

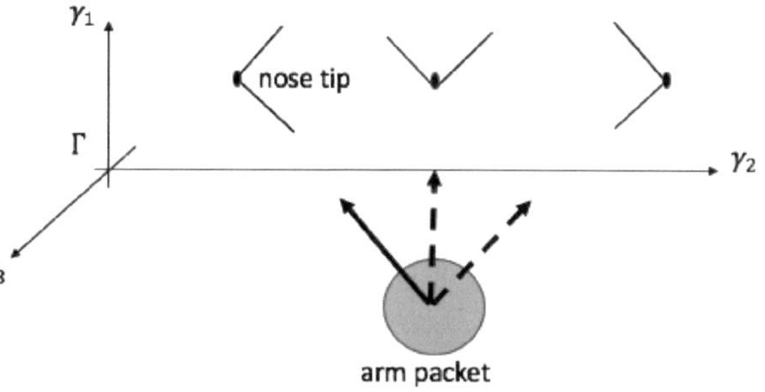

Figure 11.
Imagine raising your arm and touching the tip of your nose in three consecutive positions: looking to the left, looking straight ahead, and looking to the right. Population vector in the packet determining arm movement rotates accordingly. Coordinates of the nose tip in mental space control tuning of numerous neurons in the arm packet. Seminal studies in [51–53] demonstrated that movement organization involves rotation of packet vectors in the direction of the target.

($\sigma(T)$ is analogous to membrane potential determined by the difference in ions concentration on both sides of the membrane, $\sigma(T)$ declines as temperature grows, E_m is an inverse of MB's permeability (resistance)). Packets connected by associative links might not be mutually accessible if separated by high energy barriers, as illustrated in **Figure 12**.
The height of energy barrier E_m determines relative stability of packet X_m that corresponds, roughly, to a level of subjective confidence in X_m, which can vary depending on the local temperature (the lower the temperature, the higher the barrier. Consistent with [54], temperature variations shape the landscape and facilitate jumps of free energy barriers. Under the notion that deployment of neuronal resources serves to extract free energy from the environment [11, 12] temperate can be viewed as a control parameter regulating access to intra-packet resources, which equates temperature inverse to a cost, in entropy, of the free energy reward from the outside [54] received by the system as a result of the packet's deployment). The subjective experience of local temperature corresponds, roughly, to a level of arousal associated with object α_m. As a result, circumstances are possible when packets having low evidential support (low cumulative strength of internal associations) remain stable, separate from other packets and inaccessible to coordination with them.

2. Variations in the mode of energy delivery (level of arousal, sustained and focused attention vs. wandering and diffuse attention) cause deformations in the landscape and enable overcoming energy barriers. **Figure 13** illustrates these notions.
   Maintaining focused attention underlies the experience of cognitive effort that accompanies recall or attempts to ascertain connections between some entities (e.g., objects represented by packets X_i and X_k). The experience was best described in [56], as shown in **Figure 14**.

3. Mental models are synergistic neuronal complexes that comprise packets, regulatory neuronal structures that coordinate rotation of packet vectors, and

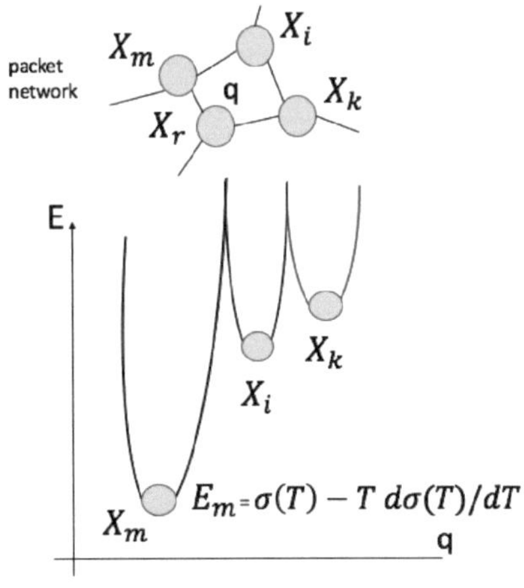

Figure 12.
Here, q denotes a coordinate in the packet network space packets X_m and X_i are adjacent in the network but are not mutually accessible due to a high energy barrier that separates them. By contrast, packets X_i and X_k are mutually accessible (think of a terrain where X_i and X_k settlements are located in the same valley and are separated by a steep hill from X_m).

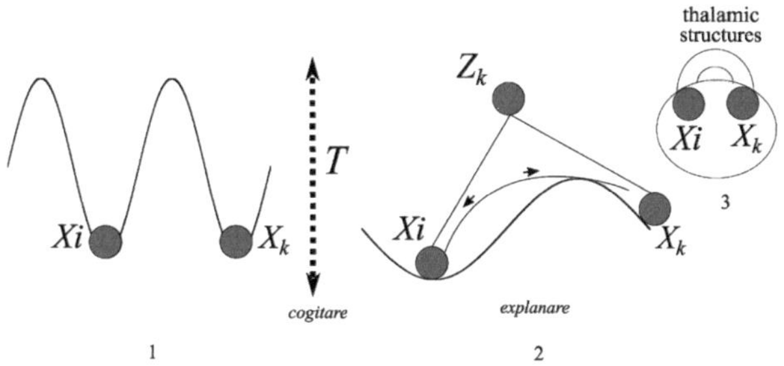

Figure 13.
1) elevated arousal combined with diffuse attention equate to increasing temperature across patches in the packet network, causing temporary lowering of energy barriers and enabling inter-packet coordination (term 'cognition' derives from the Latin cogitare*: Shaking together [55]. 2) sustained, focused attention equate to targeted energy delivery sufficient for local lowering and overcoming of the energy barriers, enabling coordination (term explanation derived from the Latin* explanare*: Flatten, make level or plane (Harper-Collins Dictionary of Philosophy, 1992). 3) inter-packet coordination can involve structures residing outside packet network (i.e., cortico-thalamo–cortical connections, vs. cortico-cortical connections).*

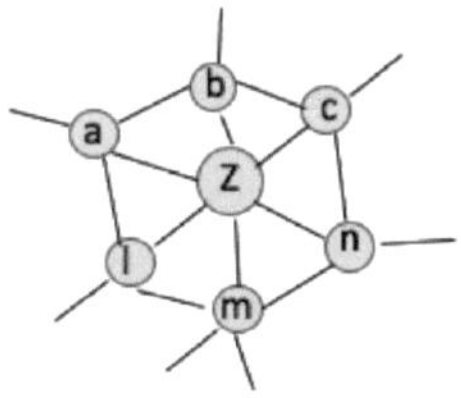

Figure 14.
The experience of mental effort. "Call the forgotten thing Z, the first facts with which we felt it was related to a, b, and c, and the details finally operative in calling it up 1, m, and n. The activity in Z will at first be a mere tension; but as the activities in a, b, and c little by little irradiate into l, m, and n ... their combined irradiations upon Z succeed in helping the tension there to overcome the resistance, and in rousing Z to full activity. Through hovering of the attention in the neighborhood of the desired object, the accumulation of associates becomes so great that the combined tensions of their neural processes break through the bar, and the nervous wave pours into the tract, which has so long been awaiting its advent" ([56] p. 586).

excitatory-inhibitory connections between the packets serving to constrain vector rotation. **Figure 15** illustrates these notions.

4. Mental modeling entered the stage (i.e., Sapience emerged) when mental processes became decoupled from the motor-sensory feedback. The hypothesis is that neuronal machinery of sensory-motor coordination richly developed in the protohuman was adopted for the task of mental coordination not accompanied by any overt activities [28]. As a result, neuronal mechanisms could retain a rich repertoire of coordination capabilities but became unencumbered by the spatio-temporal constraints facing sensory-motor acts (e.g., when raising a hand, one cannot skip over intermediate positions or exceed the range and speed limits afforded by the muscular-skeletal system. By contrast, envisioning the same act does not face such restrictions).

Decoupling from motor-sensory feedback created a gateway into mental universe populated by products of composition (imagination). To yield adaptive benefits, regulatory mechanisms were needed that would curtail superfluous compositions and facilitate those that could be mapped back onto and benefit overt behavior (i.e., allow predictions). Understanding is such a mechanism: although being rooted in sensory-motor coordination, understanding allows predictions unrestricted by spatio-temporal limitations of sensory-motor processes

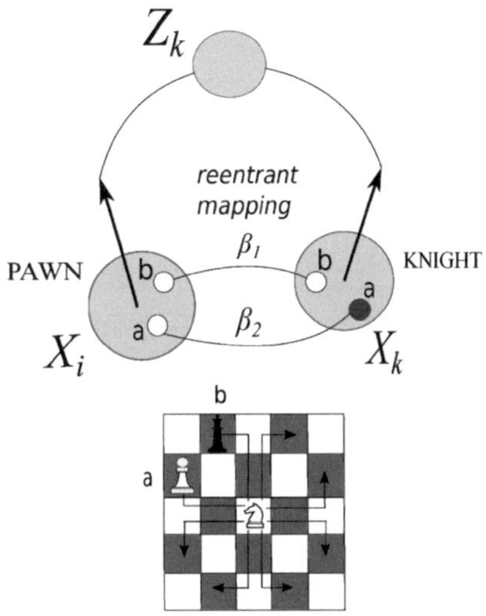

Figure 15.
*Understanding chess positions. White knight can move to 8 squares, thinking of possible moves involves consecutive activation of one place neuron and inhibiting the other seven in the knight packet. Place neuron responding to square **a** in the white pawn packet inhibits the corresponding neuron in the knight packet. As a result, the idea of moving knight to square **a** does not come to mind. Place neuron responding to square b in the knight packet excites place neuron b in the pawn packet, and vice versa. As a result, the idea of taking the black pawn by either the white pawn or the white knight presents itself prominently (one 'sees' the opportunity).*

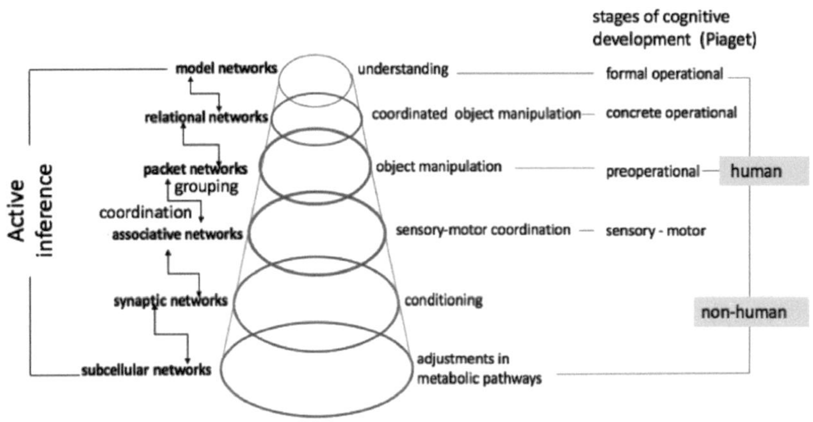

Figure 16.
Functional architecture underlying active inference. The architecture comprises 6 levels, from subcellular to model networks. Subcellular networks at the bottom coordinate movement of mitochondria and substances across cell populations and inside cells. The model network on top comprises a multitude of mental models spreading across different tasks and domains. Interactions between levels are two directional: Intra-level processes form groups of elements that are treated as (composite) elements in the next level above; in turn, upper level-processes influence conditions and coordinate groupings in the level below. The packet network plays a pivotal role in the architecture, bridging levels shared by all species and those that are unique to the humans and become operational gradually in the course of an individual's cognitive development.

or the speed of neuronal signaling. At the same time, mental models are subject to constraints of a different kind, including the explainability requirement and, crucially, limitations imposed by processes (reentrant mapping) that are inherent in the coordination mechanisms and allow eliminating superfluous degrees of freedom in the model constituents. **Figure 16** summarizes assumptions and suggestions in this part, presenting a sketch of functional hierarchy underlying active inference.

Emergence of packets underlies perception, i.e., extraction of quasi-stable, bounded feature groupings (objects) from the sensory stream (e.g., one can discern and subsequently recognize different chess pieces). The relational level is split in two – behavioral and relational proper. In the former, different behavior patterns are attributed to the objects (e.g., admissible moves are defined for knight, as in **Figure 15**). In the latter, inter-object relations get decoupled from the objects' sensory contents (e.g., coordinations in **Figure 15** make no account of the shape, color, weight, etc. of the participating pieces). Finally, operations in the model network support mental experiments (gedanken experiments) – a form of active inference most distant from the control of motor-sensory feedback. Mental experiments can entail physical experiments but do not rely on them in assessing assess the validity of their conclusions.

Ideas and suggestions in this section do not answer questions **a** and **b** posed at the end of Section 2 but, arguably, indicate directions for further inquiry. Question **c** will be addressed briefly in the discussion. The ideas are speculative, the next section references findings and theories in the literature that seem to agree with the ideas and might help assessing their biological plausibility.

4.3 Assessing plausibility

A thumbnail summary of the preceding two sections: Cognitive processes yield adaptive behavior via two regulatory loops: the first loop optimizes (coordinates) deployment of sensory-motor resources while the second loop coordinates deployment of neuronal resources. The first loop produces associative networks that give rise to packet networks, the second loop combines packets into nested coordinated structures (mental models). The second loop was decoupled from the motor-sensory feedback, which created an opportunity for constructing unlimited multitudes of mental models. Realization of that opportunity was predicated on satisfying two constraints: a) using a limited number of neurons and b) maintaining energy consumption below some physiologically attainable thresholds. It can be shown that mechanisms of packets and packet coordination are deployment heuristics serving to satisfy the constraints [11, 12]. Packet coordination underlies understanding, which is a form of active inference unique to Sapience. The remainder of this section references findings supporting key notions in this proposal.

4.3.1 Tuning neuronal resources

Dynamic allocation of neuronal resources implies that neurons have a degree of plasticity, i.e. their receptive fields (RF) can be changed by both the stimuli and, crucially, brain systems that regulate allocation. A body of findings in [57–62] provide ample evidence of such plasticity, including stimulus-driven adaptive plasticity, rapid attention-driven plasticity, and consolidated learning-induced plasticity. Rapid attention-driven plasticity manifests in attentional modulation of neuronal processes and underlies the ability of the brain to make coordinated changes in stimuli-driven and self-directed neuronal activities as the context and task demands change. "These transformations occur at the level of synapses, single-neuron RFs, and also at the level of brain networks" ([63] p. 252).

4.3.2 Optimizing deployment of neuronal resources

The idea to characterize cognitive processes as resource optimization has been explored repeatedly in several forms, as optimization of energetic resources [64], optimization of computing resources [65], optimization of cognitive resources [66]. The present theory characterizes cognition as deployment of neuronal resources optimized for energy efficiency, under an exceedingly simple model ("neurons fire at stimuli"): successful allocation of neurons to streaming stimuli procures energy deposits from the stimuli and incurs energy costs (recruiting, firing, maintaining neurons), neuronal system seeks to maximize the former while minimizing the latter [12]. It can be shown that, under this model, elements of functional architecture in **Figure 16** represent heuristics delivering progressively improving energy inflows while reducing energy costs (optimal maneuvering of neuronal resources to maximize gains and minimize losses). Other major phenomena can be mapped straightforwardly onto the model, e.g. in the context of resource optimization, the short term memory/long term memory partitioning turns out to be a powerful heuristic involving breaking large optimization problems into successions of small ones thus cutting down the amount of computation while keeping the outcome in the vicinity of global optimum. Optimal allocation strategies include prediction and anticipatory recruitment (active inference), combining those with cost minimization enabled expansion and diversification of inference domains. Dynamic resource optimization requires unencumbered access to all resources in the resource pool and flexible switching between resource groupings. These notions resonate with proposals in the literature, some examples follow.

A model in [67] postulates a global workspace composed of distributed and heavily interconnected neurons, and a set of specialized modules conducting perceptual, motor, evaluative, and attentional operations. Workspace (regulatory) neurons are mobilized in effortful tasks and selectively mobilize or suppress, through descending connections, the contribution of specific processor neurons. When workspace neurons become spontaneously co- activated, they form spatio-temporal patterns that are subject to modulation by vigilance signals.

The idea of cost-reward tradeoffs is consistent with the findings in [68]. This study examined neuronal substrate responsible for balancing expected performance rewards and their cognitive costs. Single-unit recordings in monkeys provided evidence that neurons in Medial Frontal Cortex (MFC) encode associations between action sets and their rewarding values and are involved in the cost- reward tradeoffs. MFC evaluates the costs incurred in executing cognitively demanding tasks and the expected gains, and recruits control resources in the Lateral Prefrontal Cortex (LPC) as necessary for compensating performance costs. MFC responses also reflect intrinsic MFC processes inhibiting inappropriate behaviors and energizing the LPC resources involved in selecting alternative behaviors according to the rewards and penalties at stake. The ideas concerning the cost-reward tradeoffs are consistent with those in [69].

The overall notion of dynamically optimized recruitment of neuronal resources is consistent with findings in [70] associating competent performance across multiple domains ("general intelligence") with selective recruitment of lateral frontal cortex in one or both hemispheres. These same frontal regions were found to be recruited by a broad range of cognitive demands, thus suggesting that "general intelligence" derives from flexibly switching recruitment between different neuronal groups. Another facet of neuronal processes implicit in the idea of neuronal resource optimization is "neuronal reuse", i.e. engaging the same circuitry for different behavioral purposes [71]. Combining quasi-stable neuronal packets without changing the packets or the underlying mosaic of associative links is a form of reuse. Improving energy efficiency can be a factor in the optimization of cerebral cortex layout and physical embedding of processing networks in the brain volume [72]): minimization of total connection length [73] reduces energy costs of signal propagation.

4.3.3 Improving energy efficiency

Neuronal processes consume significant amount of energy, consumption increases with activity which demands local and global changes in metabolic rates and blood flow. Mechanisms of efficiency and energy transduction in the brain have been investigated in numerous studies [74–78]. Energy is produced through oxygen consumption mediated by the mitochondrial respiratory chain generating the high-energy phosphorous metabolite (adenosine triphosphate, or ATP). The carbon source that supports the oxidative metabolism is predominantly glucose. About 20% of the total oxygen consumption in the body takes place in the brain. A detailed account of energy consumption was obtained in a recent study utilizing ^{31}P-MRS in vivo imaging of the human brain [79]. It was determined that approximately 5.7 kg of ATP molecules is produced and utilized by the cortical gray and white matter in a day, which is equivalent to the complete oxidative combustion of 56 g glucose per day and is almost five times the total weight of the gray and white matter ($\approx$1.2 kg). The energy expenditure of a single cortical neuron is 4.7 billion ATPs per second (compared than 3.3 billion ATPs/neuron/sec estimated for the rat brain). Approximately 67–75% of the total energy expenditures is used for neurotransmitter signaling and electrophysiological activities involved in sustaining neuronal functions [79].

It has been long recognized that the high energetic cost of human brain function, which is 10 times higher than what would be expected from its weight alone, can only be maintained through efficient energy use [80, 81]. Accordingly, theories were advanced suggesting that brains evolved to be metabolically efficient [82–84] which implies that representations of events and actions should be sculpted to involve as few action potentials and active synapses as possible. For optimum efficiency, less than 4% of a population of cortical neurons should be activated to represent a new event. Neural mechanisms associated with attention restrict the volume of cortex in which activity is elevated [85]. The arrangements of neuronal systems are thought to allow maximum communication speed with minimal energy expenditures [86].

Massive data was accumulated demonstrating reduction of metabolic costs in the organization of motor performance and regulation of movement economy [87–93]. As noted in [94], metabolic determinants of physical action organization might not be the same as those determining cognitive action organization. However, it stands to reason to assume that the principle of cost minimization applies in both domains.

Analysis in [85] concludes that strategies directed at maximizing metabolic efficiency are indeed used by the brain. In particular, a) fine axon collaterals reduce the number of ions required to transmit an action potential, by reducing membrane area, b) the arrangement of neurons in maps reduces the distance the potentials must travel and c) sparse codes reduce the number of action potentials required to represent events. **Figure 17** indicates that suggestions in the present theory resonate with those formulated in [85] and other studies.

4.3.4 Neuronal packets are building blocks in cognitive processes

The idea that dynamically formed neuronal groupings (assemblies, ensembles) are the basic functional units in neuronal processes was advanced by [95] and subsequently developed in the Theory of Neuronal Group Selection (TNGS) by Gerald Edelman [96–98] and explored in other studies. For example, [99] suggests that acquisition of motor skills involves development of motor primitives amenable to adaptive re-combination (arguably, motor primitives are rooted in the underlying neuronal assemblies), [100] conceptualizes mental synthesis as a synchronization of independent neuronal ensembles, etc. Hebb's idea received experimental support in a number of recent findings: studies in [86, 101] demonstrated existence of neuronal assemblies entering into different combinations as the tasks and conditions change. Assemblies observed in [86] comprise a few dozen neurons each and can

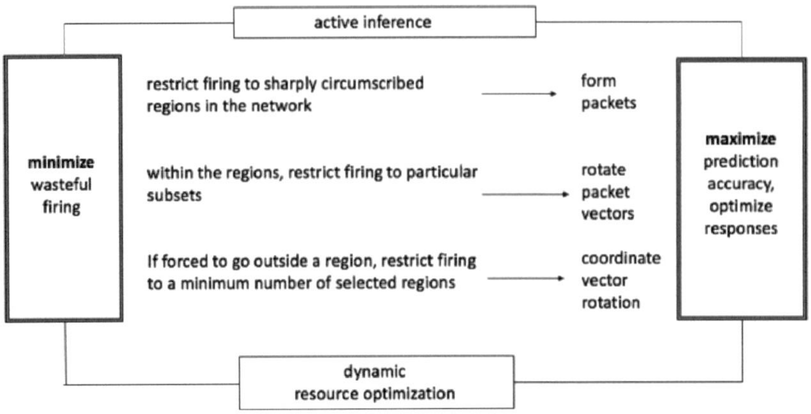

Figure 17.
Connected associative network allows unrestricted signal propagation, i.e., excitation of any neuron can ignite excitation spreading that will, eventually, engulf the entire network. Formation of packets and operations on them minimize spreading, confining excitation to the smallest subset of neurons producing the largest expected energy gain. Dynamic resource optimization boils down to suppressing wasteful firing and facilitating beneficial firing, i.e. yielding maximum prediction accuracy and response composition optimal under the prediction. In that sense, resource optimization is an engine of active inference.

be interlaced within the same volume. It was suggested that "elementary neuronal groups are prescribed Lego-like building blocks of perception and that acquired memory relies on combining these elementary assemblies into higher-order constructs" [86]. Both studies suggest that their findings reveal a synaptic organizing principle (i.e., grouping) that is common across animals.

An important elaboration of the notion of assembly received in the idea of *synergistic structural units* formulated in [102–106]. Synergistic structural units can be combined into task- specific groupings and, crucially, are amenable to "nonindividualized control", that is, their constituent elements can be controlled by a few task-related variables (goals) [103].

The notion of 'neuronal packets' builds on the idea of Hebbian assembly and is consistent with the finding and suggestion referenced above. However, the notion offers two crucial extensions to the idea, as follows: a) neuronal packets form as a result of phase transition in associative networks causing some subnets to fold into cohesive units (packets) and b) folding establishes energy barriers at the packet boundaries. Stated differently, boundary energy barriers implement Markov blankets separating packet internals from the surrounding network [30]. More precisely, the height of energy barriers equals free energy per unit of surface area (surface tension) determined by the total membrane surface in the packet's boundary neurons (i.e., packet's Markov blanket, see **Figure 9**). Analysis in [85] identified reduction of membrane areas in individual neurons as a factor contributing into brain's metabolic efficiency. In a similar way, thermodynamically-driven tendency to minimize packet surface areas [27] contributes to the metabolic efficiency of neuronal processes (see **Figure 17**).

4.3.5 Coordinated rotation of packet vectors

Phase transitions transform groups of associated neurons into cohesive functional units amenable to synergistic control and re-combination with other units (reuse). The present theory defines coordinated rotation of packet vectors as a form of synergistic control, extending control mechanism described in [51–53, 107–111] from controlling overt movements to controlling mental 'movements' (i.e., packet vector rotation and coordination, see **Figure 15**). This generalization is consistent

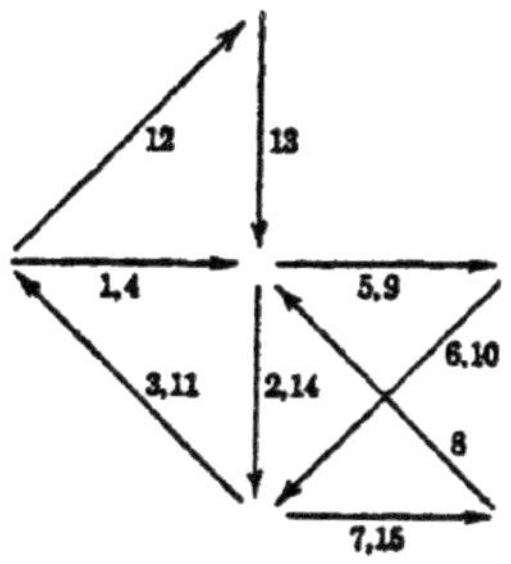

Figure 18.
Neuronal assemblies were conceptualized as complex structures affording different trajectories for excitation propagation (adopted from [95]).

with the original concept of neuronal assemblies in [95] envisioning the possibility of the assemblies producing different responses constituted by different excitation trajectories within the assembly, as shown in **Figure 18**.

The notion of packet vector trajectories appears to be consistent with the findings in [112] demonstrating that memorization involves formation of specific sequences of spike bursts in the cortex that are replayed during retrieval. The function of coordination (neurons Z_k in **Figure 15**) can be carried out by components of basal ganglia, thalamus and other structures. In particular, [113] suggests that basal ganglia chunks the representations of motor and cognitive action sequences so that they can be implemented as performance units. Studies in [114] uncovered activities in basal ganglia circuits that encoded sequences as single actions. Besides start/stop signaling and sequence parsing, these neurons displayed inhibited or sustained activity throughout the execution of the sequences. This sustained activity co-varied with the rate of execution of individual sequence elements, consistent with motor concatenation. Direct and indirect pathways of basal ganglia were concomitantly active during sequence initiation, but behaved differently during performance. Thalamic relays also play a critical role in coordination [115, 116]. The cerebellum is also involved in the detection and generation of sequences [117].

Cortical coordination and dynamics have been analyzed in [118–121] concluding that "the formation of neural context through the coordinated mutual constraint of multiple interacting cortical areas, is considered as a guiding principle underlying all cognitive functions" ([120] p. 140). The present theory agrees with that conclusion and suggests neuronal mechanisms instantiating the idea. In particular, the theory defines mental models as tightly coordinated gestalts, or *structural units* where changes in one component cause reciprocal changes in the other ones (e.g. when one hand is used to lift a heavy object from a tray supported by the other hand, increasing effort in one hand is concomitant with relaxation in the other one – hands form a structural unit (Gelfand et al). The same coordination mechanism underlies operation of mental models, e. g, in a catapult model, increasing distance to the target entails the realization that projectile need to be shifted in the opposite direction). The modeling mechanisms includes coordinated vector rotation and reentrant mapping.

4.3.6 Reentrant mapping

The hypothesis that reentrant signaling serves as a general mechanism to facilitate the coordination of neuronal firing in anatomically and functionally segregated cortical areas and in the thalamus is one of the main tenets in the Theory of Neuronal Groups Selection (TNGS) [122–124]. According to TNGS, neurons belonging to different cortical areas are reciprocally interconnected by reentrant networks of excitatory axons, and each cortical area is also reentrantly interconnected by large numbers of axons to one or more nuclei of the thalamus. These thalamocortical and cortico-thalamic reentrant connections modulate brain arousal and help determining which of the patterns of environmental signals arriving in the thalamus from the environment will be relayed on to the cortex. They also participate in the execution of timed, sequential, or willed processes, such as manipulating mental constructs, or issuing segmented motor commands [124]. The present theory is consistent with TNGS principles, making reentrant mapping (or bidirectional coupling [113]) integral to the mechanisms of modeling and understanding (see **Figure 15**).

4.3.7 Energy landscapes – a missing link in cognitive neuroscience

It has been long recognized that the concept on neuronal assembly leaves the issues of stability and borders undetermined (how does the brain 'know' where one assembly ends and another begins, how does a neuron 'know' to which assembly it belongs, what keeps neurons in an assembly together, etc.)? In the original conceptualization [95], waves of excitations develop and reverberate inside assemblies - this notion indicates intuition of assembly borders but that intuition was not made explicit. The original conceptualization in [95] entailed a possibility that activity in any assembly will spread to other assemblies and ultimately to the entire cortex or even the total brain, resulting in pathological overactivity, as in seizures. To cope with the problem, the idea of a "threshold control mechanism" was introduced [125] with the subsequent elaborations placing the mechanism in the basal ganglia or the hippocampus. The idea was that a cell assembly "holds" at a threshold θ when at that threshold all the neurons of the assembly, once excited, stay active due to their reciprocal excitatory connections. Manipulation of the thresholds was envisioned as follows (compare to **Figure 13**(1)).

> *"A periodic operation (colloquially called the "pump of thoughts") may involve the following steps. Given a certain input I, the threshold is lowered so that the set of active neurons FI will go over into a larger set F'I. This will encourage the ignition of cell assemblies. As the threshold is again raised, activity is smothered and only the most strongly connected cell assembly will survive. A new cycle beginning again with a lowered threshold will bring in new cell assemblies. They may include an even more strongly connected cell assembly, which will be the next one to survive when the threshold is raised. The evolution will be in the direction of the most strongly connected cell assemblies.... One may express this by saying that the system hunts for an interpretation of the input, or that it 'thinks" ([125] p.177).*

Independently from the proposal in [125], the idea of threshold regulation was advanced in a theory of movement coordination (λ theory) in [126–128] According to λ theory theory, coordination of motor actions involves centrally controlled resetting of the threshold positions of body segments. Deviations from the threshold positions (e.g., restive muscle length) trigger resistive forces, detection of differences between the centrally set threshold positions and the sensory-signaled actual positions cause activation of neuromuscular elements seeking to diminish the difference. The crucial assumption is that thresholds are changed by descending fibers that influence membrane potentials of motoneurons in motor cortices, either directly or via interneurons [126].

Arguably, theories of threshold regulation [125, 126] are motivated by intuition similar to that expressed in **Figures 13-15**. In the present theory, boundary barriers are an intrinsic property of neuronal assemblies (packets), regulation of barrier height involves changes in membrane potential in neurons residing in the packet's MB. Boundary energy barriers make assemblies distinct, quasi-stable and immersed in energy landscapes. The landscape curtails activation spreading, by imposing energy costs on inter-assembly transitions.

More precisely, the present theory postulates that boundary barriers establish energy landscapes across packet networks [10, 12]. Accordingly, formation of packets can be viewed as a form of folding, analogous to the folding of proteins and other complex molecular structures [129–131]. As in proteins, the folding of packets is a spontaneous process obtaining stable (equilibrium) configurations of minimal free energy [27]. Stability is maintained within some ranges of temperature variation (packets dissolve when $\sigma(T) \approx T\, d\sigma(T)/dT$, $E_m \to 0$, the constituent neurons become absorbed into the surrounding packets). Within the multidimensional energy surface, packets' Markov Blankets and the corresponding cutsets (links connecting MB to the surrounding packets) form attraction basins in the neighborhood of local minima, connected by saddle points. As a result, attentive navigation of the landscape involves energy-demanding (effortful) basin-to-basin transitions. Deformations in the energy landscape determine changes in the accessibility of neuronal packets. Presumably, transitions are controlled by frontal /prefrontal networks and thalamic structures.

A number of experimental results appear to agree with the proposal. Findings in [132] demonstrating fast transitions between separated states of cortical activity involving distinct neuronal groups appear to agree with above proposal. Findings in [133] indicate that thalamic cells respond selectively to complex percepts and concepts conferred on them by the cortical assemblies in whose activation they participate. The cortico-thalamo-cortical pathways provide connections between different cortical loci which have higher reliability than the direct cortico-cortical routes, and play crucial role in orchestrating activation of those assemblies). Important findings in [134] demonstrated that brain network are structured in a manner optimized for network control, which includes increased controllability and reduced synchronizability (controllability characterizes the ease of switching from one dynamical state to another, traversing energy landscape (see Figure 130; synchronizability characterizes the ability for regions in the network to support the same temporal dynamical patterns).

The idea of energy landscapes in brain systems remained purely speculative until the recent pioneering studies in [135–137] applied modern analytic and modeling techniques (e.g. network disconnectivity analysis) to fMRI data, seeking to define energy landscapes in Default Mode Network (DMN) and Fronto Parietal Network (FPN). It was determined that DMN energy landscape consisted of two groups of low-energy local minima that are separated by a relatively high energy barrier. Within each group, the activity patterns of the local minima were similar, and different minima were connected by relatively low energy barriers. In the FPN, all dominant local minima were separated by relatively low energy barriers such that they formed a single coarse-grained global minimum. The height of energy barriers separating local minima influences the rate of inter-state transitions. Accordingly, transitions in DNM occur at a low rate while transitions between local minima in FPN occur more easily. The notion that brain operates at the edge of instability and transits between low energy states has been explored in multiple studies [50, 138]). It appears that the notion of brain energy landscapes was introduced in [10, 12], and experimental mapping of energy landscapes was attempted for the first time in [136].

To summarize, the folding of subnets in associative networks forms packets separated by Markov Blankets from the rest of the network. Packet Markov Blankets are constituted by boundary energy barriers that make packets distinct, quasi-stable

stable (i.e., amenable to modification but at substantial energy cost) and synergistic (i.e. amenable to control by a few variables and coordination with other packets). Boundary barriers establishes energy landscapes across packet networks and determine both kinematic (inter-packet transitions) and dynamic properties of neuronal organization.

4.3.8 Accommodations

It was suggested that lateral inhibition prevents neuronal assemblies from encroaching on each other while the tendency towards reducing surface tension in the packets favors their coalescence (minimizing the amount of free energy in the surface). Arguably, the interplay of the opposite tendencies drives 'accommodation', that is, spontaneous adjustments inside the neuronal systems following changes resulting from interactions with the environment [27].

The notions of assimilation, accommodation and cognitive equilibration were introduced in [18] denoting, correspondingly, integration of new information into the existing structures, re-organization of those structures, until a state of equilibrium is reached obtaining a sufficient degree of integration via a minimal amount of structural changes. According to the present theory, assimilation involves changes in the distribution of synaptic weights, that trigger waves of packet re-structuring propagating throughout the packet network (the accommodation). In this way, the requirement of spontaneous re-structuring is inherent in the notion of neuronal packets immersed in energy landscapes. On that view, the overall functional architecture of the cognitive systems was reduced to three modules: associative cortices, reticular formation controlling arousal level, and a frontal/prefrontal module controlling landscape navigation. Accommodation and assimilation are confined to packet networks [10].

Recent experimental findings and theoretical proposals [139] envision functional architecture comprising Default Mode Network (DMN) [140], Salience Network (SN) [141] and Task Control Network (TCN) [142], as follows. A DMN is a large network comprises hubs in medial prefrontal cortex, posterior cingulate/ precuneus and angular gyrus becomes active under conditions of wakeful rest, i.e. when person is not engaged in any task. The SN comprises a suite of brain regions whose cortical hubs are the anterior cingulate and ventral anterior insular cortices while the TCN (a cingulo-opercular task-control network) is anchored in the dorsal anterior insula and the frontal operculum. SN detects behaviorally relevant stimuli and recruits neural resources to orchestrate responses. For the latter, the SN engages the TCN (or Central Executive) whose functions include maintaining relevant task set or orchestrate switching to a new task set in response to shifts in the salience landscape.

Significantly, a comprehensive study in [143] compared functional networks in the brain during task performance (active brain) and at rest (resting brain), concluding that the full repertoire of functional networks utilized in active brain (Active Brain Networks, or ABN) remains continuously active in the resting brain (Resting State Networks, or RSN, including the "default mode network"). The study applied independent component analysis (ICA) and other modern techniques to two sets of fMRI functional imaging data: "active brain" data in the BrainMap data base collected from over 30,000 subjects, and resting brain data collected from 36 subjects. The ICA decomposition was conducted at two resolution levels, 20-component analysis and 70-component analysis, with the higher resolution analysis revealing subnetworks in the primary networks determined at the lower resolution level. It was found that primary networks split into subnetworks in both active and resting data in almost identical ways, maintaining greater functional (temporal) correlation between subnetworks within a primary network than across primary networks. Analysis in both levels produced converging results: close to 70% overlap in the composition of Active State Network and Resting State Networks. The analysis concludes with an admission: "Although we have shown that activation networks are mirrored in resting data, we must acknowledge that this does not begin to answer the question of why the brain's many regions continue to "function" (with large amplitude fluctuations) when the subject is at rest, and even when the subject is asleep and under anesthesia" [143].

It appears that these findings are consistent with the proposal in [10] envisioning waves of accommodating adjustments in packet networks. Moreover, the adjustment requirements are inherent in the notion of packet networks. In particular, the hypothesis is that variations in temperature and synaptic weight distribution across packet networks cause changes in the resting membrane potentials [144] in the MB neurons, thus creating potential gradients in the packet network causing adjustments in the energy landscape and re-distribution of neurons seeking packet configurations in the vicinity of global energy minima. Stated differently, energy landscape is "frustrated" [131] due to conflicting tendencies of lateral inhibition and lateral coalescence. Spontaneous re-organizations in packet networks to resolve frustration move the system in the direction of cognitive equilibrium. Possibly, neuronal avalanches are a form of such re-organization, playing a role in maintaining network stability and preventing runaway excitation [145]. **Figure 19** makes suggestions regarding the placement of packet networks in the tri-partite architecture [139, 146].

Figure 19 suggests that DMN/SN/CEN interplay focuses on the engagement of prefrontal areas in coordination activities, i.e., formation of relations and operations on relational networks. Accordingly, it can be expected that prefrontal damages are likely to cause severe deficits in integration of relations. The order of operation in the DMN/SN/CEN system is, roughly, as follows: a) the Central Executive Network includes the agency of attention and controls attention focusing and other processes engaged in the performance of cognitive tasks, b) the Default Mode Network becomes active when the person remains awake but no tasks are pursued, c) the Salience Network administers switching between CEN and DMN.

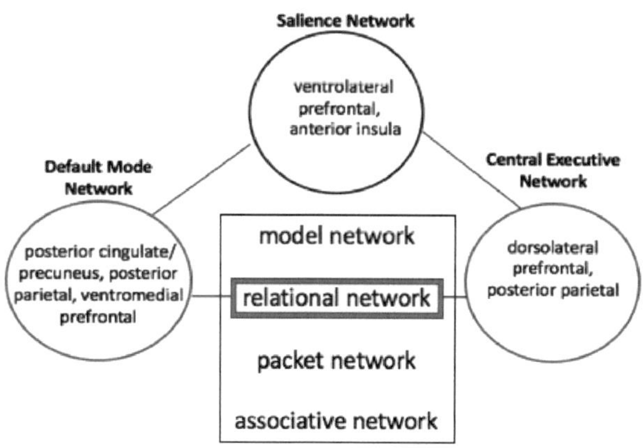

Figure 19.
Operations on networks underlying understanding capacity involve an interplay between default mode network and central executive network (CEN). Salience network coordinates switching between DMN and CEN [146]. This general architecture allows more detailed mapping onto anatomical structures in the brain underlying functional organization [147–149].

4.3.9 Decoupling

The present theory attributes emergence of human understanding to evolutionary developments causing decoupling of regulatory processes from the sensory-motor feedback loops [10, 28]. The idea is consistent with suggestions in [150] regarding evolutionary origins of human cognition. Analysis [150] focuses on the development of cerebral cortex, pointing at its vast expansion in the humans relative to other primates (the cerebral surface area is 120 cm^2 in the macaque and 960 cm^2 in the human) and disproportionate expansion of distributed association regions within the cortex. The hypothesis is that rapid expansion of the cortical mantle may have decoupled ("untethered") large portions of the cortex from sensory hierarchies and resulted in the development of networks that either control processes in the sensory networks or are engaged in parallel activities that are "detached from sensory perception and motor actions – what one might term 'internal mentation" [150].

5. Discussion and conclusions

In a letter to Nature Neuroscience entitled "What does 'understanding' mean"?, the author confesses that "upon reflection, it is depressing, if not scandalous, to realize how rarely I ask myself this" [151]. Arguably, the letter's intent was not to confess ignorance or lack of interest but to point out that a critically important issue has been long neglected. There is nothing that one is familiar more intimately and directly with than sensations of confusion, mental effort and understanding (except, perhaps, for the sensations of one's own breathing and heart beating), yet the issue of understanding has not been receiving significant attention in cognitive sciences (see some discussion in [27, 152]). The intent of this chapter was to suggest that a theory of understanding might be within reach (and grasp), requiring the synthesis of new ideas and the long existing ones, re-evaluated in the light of new data. The proposed theoretical framework is that of active inference [13, 14] carried out under the requirements of limited neuronal pool size and minimized energy expenditures. Within that framework, the meaning of 'understanding' reduces to optimization strategy in the deployment of neuronal resources that enables expanding domains of inference while minimizing expansion costs. In subjective experiences, the meaning of understanding reduces to attaining 'grasp', i.e. unifying some disparate entities, in a coordinated relational structure that enables relational [153, 154] and other forms of reasoning. Attaining 'grasp' can be accompanied by cognitive strain and culminates in exhilaration and euphoria making the activity self-rewarding (the Greek *euporia* stands for 'easy passage or travel' while its opposite *aporia* denotes 'difficulty or impossibility of passage' [48]). This section will compare the present proposal to some findings in the literature, aiming to suggest directions for further research.

5.1 Mental simulations

The phenomenon of mental modeling (mental simulations) has been addressed in a number of studies [155–157], focusing on the "paradox" of endogenously-driven mental activity:" how can findings that carry conviction result from a new experiment conducted entirely within the head" [155]. Data has been accumulated demonstrating that mental simulations engage mechanisms that are different from those involved in reasoning based on descriptive knowledge, exhibit analogue properties, and can produce correct inferences when descriptive knowledge is lacking. At the same time, it was observed that mental simulations proceed in a piecemeal fashion (not a holistic image) [157].

The present proposal pivots on the notion that mental modeling was made possible by decoupling regulatory processes from the motor-sensory feedback, which shifted the power of conviction from experiments in the world to experiments in the head (e.g., arguments in Pythagorean theorem are entirely convincing but not amenable to experimental verification). On the account of the present theory, the experience of understanding accompanies formation of tightly coordinated gestalts which, simultaneously, afford some degrees of freedom to their constituents. Exploring these degrees of freedom can indeed proceed in a step-by-step fashion, i.e. experimental findings in [157] and are not incompatible with the theory. Other proposals in the recent literature addressing the role of mental simulation [158] resonate with the key notions in this theory.

5.2 Transient assemblies and the searchlight hypothesis

The operation of focused attention was compared to a searchlight that shifts between and thus helps forming conjunctions of separate attributes or features of perceived objects [159]. It was further proposed that functions of the "searchlight" are carried out by activity bursts in thalamic nuclei while conjunctions are implemented by rapidly modifiable synapses (called Malsburg synapses), orchestrated by the bursts to produce transient cell assemblies [160].

Notwithstanding suggestions in [159, 160] concerning transient assemblies, considering the role of focused attention in manipulating quasi-stable assemblies (packets) calls for a different metaphor. A neuronal packet is a superposition of multiple behavior patterns afforded by an object. Overcoming energy barrier and shifting attention from outside the packet to the inside (see **Figure 13**(2)) actualizes one of the patterns. Think of 'grasp' as seizing an object and holding it in a closed fist, followed by opening the fist and holding the object in an open palm. With the eyes closed, one needs to run the fingertip of another hand over the object in order to discern its shape. The point is that concentrating attention amounts to focusing energy delivery on particular neurons causing their excitation or inhibition, which gives rise to the experience of a behaving object. In short, both the searchlight and the fingertip metaphors define attention as physical actions applied to neurons. However, the former metaphor conjures up an image of a wandering light beam falling on the elements of neuronal structures and thus making them discernable to the "mind's eye" while the latter one connotes the image of a finger (or stick) 'tapping' on the neurons, which seems to better represent the notion of physical action.

5.3 Understanding and language

The discovery of mirror neurons inspired hopes that understanding of the origins of language can be "within our grasp" [161] Mirror neurons discharge during active movements of the hand or mouth (or both) performed by the subject or observed being performed by others (hence, the mirror neurons). It was hypothesized that the latter feature establishes a bridge from 'doing' to 'communicating', or from acting to message sending [161, 162]. Other hypothesis concerning language origins attribute its emergence to internal, as opposed to communicative, functions [35–37] and conceptualize language mechanisms as the manipulation of neuronal assemblies [163, 164]. This theory offers an opinion that seems to unify all three hypotheses, as follows.

First, note that mirror neurons were determined to be of three types: 'grasping with the hand' neurons, 'holding' neurons and 'tearing' neurons [161]. Apply these notions to manipulation of mental 'objects' (as opposed to physical ones) and assume that 'grasping with the hand' denotes formation of a packet, 'holding' denotes the state when attention is "hovering outside" the packet (see **Figure 14**), and 'tearing' denotes entering the packet and experiencing the contents. A reversible 'holding' – 'tearing' transition corresponds to set operation: a manifold of features is experienced as a unity (one object) devoid of (separated from) any sensory contents, followed by experiencing a series of sensory features comprised in the object.

Next, think of watching a play performed on the stage, and then consider the same play being read to you. In the latter case, assume that the cast of characters and all the names have been removed so only the text proper remained. It is not hard to realize that figuring out what is going on might be possible but extremely difficult, requiring forming and comparing different word combinations (e.g. "The queen, my lord, is dead. She should have died hereafter..." – who is talking here? Note that you are facing no such challenges when watching the play). Finally, imagine that only the cast of characters and names are extracted from the text and the rest is discarded. Clearly, it can be very hard but possible to make some sense of the former version while the latter one makes no sense at all. It is also evident that the range of understanding in the former version will be restricted to a few characters and a few consecutive episodes, with the text becoming an impenetrable mess after that. Restoring the original text (putting the names back where they belong) resolves the otherwise insurmountable difficulty. Here comes a tentative proposal:

Emergence of language followed decoupling from the sensory-motor feedback while retaining the mechanisms of sensory-motor coordination. Language emerged as a means to support mental coordination over an expanding variety of mental objects, by adopting the mechanisms of communicative signaling and re-purposing them for self-signaling (communicative signals make an animal aware of a predator or other condition without direct sensory confirmation of that condition). Symbols (labels) are implemented as neuronal assembles [163, 164] or 'symbol packets' attached to 'object packets', 'symbol packets' have no sensory content except for the minimum required for making them distinct. Symbols make one roughly aware of the contents of a packet without the expense of entering and examining these contents, thus facilitating landscape navigation (think of labels attached to drawers that need to be pulled with effort). The process of thinking alternates reversibly between the packet arrays (roughly, between words and images and actions they signify). Understanding phrases involves syntactic coordination and, crucially, substantive, or grounded [165] coordination (i.e., between the objects and activities signified by the words). Findings in [166] demonstrating "grasping ideas with the motor system", i.e. activation of the motor cortex by words referring to bodily actions, even idiomatically, other results [167] appear to support these contentions.

5.4 Cognitive disorders

Pathological malfunctions in the operation of the DMN/SN/CEN system (**Figure 19**) can cause breakdowns in the regulation of energy landscapes (energy barriers are rigid and remain abnormally high or abnormally low), entailing a range of cognitive disorders. In particular, abnormally high barriers hamper correlation between cortical areas and interactions between frontal and parietal, neostriatum, and thalamic areas involved in attention control, which can manifest in performance impairments characteristic of the autism spectrum disorders [168–170]. By contrast, abnormally low barriers entail destabilization and disintegration of neuronal packets, leading to irreversible memory losses and other impairments characteristic of the Alzheimer's – type disorders (e.g., subjects can be expected to fail clock drawing tests due to the inability to recollect proper elements and/or their respective positions [171]. In general, abnormally high energy barriers degrade functional connectivity between memory elements (percepts, concepts) while abnormally low barriers degrade the elements. It appears possible to relate a variety of cognitive disorders (e.g. different forms and stages of dementia) to persistent abnormalities in energy landscapes, which can potentially lead to new insights and unified approaches in the diagnosis and treatment.

To conclude, this chapter suggested a hand-in-glove relationship between an information-theoretic account of cognitive processes (active inference) and a thermodynamics-centered account asserting that neuronal mechanisms underlying active inference are sculpted by physical conditions in the brain limiting its volume and energy supply. Active inference has been conceptualized as a regulatory process allowing organisms to operate within the sensory-motor feedback loop. This is accomplished by forming generative models that anticipate consequences of overt actions as those are reflected in the sensory inflows, followed by adjustments that reconcile the actions and the models in a manner serving to satisfy the survival and other needs. This chapter applied the active inference framework to define regulatory mechanisms decoupled from the motor-sensory feedback loop, under the notion of energy-minimizing deployment of neuronal resources.

Advanced theoretical analysis seeking to unite conceptual foundations of the physical sciences and biology is uncovering a profound unity of the information-theoretic and thermodynamics-centered viewpoints, spanning the range from inanimate matter to the most complex life forms [172]. Moreover, recent experimental findings demonstrate the possibility of information-to-energy conversion [173]. Analysis indicates that self-organization obtains access to progressively higher degrees of order and organization in the channels of energy transduction [172]. The notion of increasing levels of coordination in the brain functional architecture, from subcellular processes to mental modeling, appears to agree with this general principle. Evolutionary climb to the upper reaches of organization manifested in creative thinking was made possible by minimizing energy costs in every step. On the present theory, active inference is the result and expression of that underlying, thermodynamically- enforced frugality.

In machine intelligence, the bulk of effort has been concentrated on learning techniques derived from the perceptron idea (conditioning). This proposal suggests advancing from machine learning to machine understanding, requiring a different conceptual foundation. It has been argued that human understanding requires awareness, and physical processes in the brain that evoke awareness might not be amenable to computational simulation [174]. Notwithstanding these arguments, it appears possible to construct artifacts possessing a level of understanding that does not reach human heights but exceeds those accessible to the conventional technology.

It feels appropriate to end this chapter by giving credit to those whose foresight brought them long ago to conclusions similar to those expressed here:

> *"It is worth while to speculate about cell assemblies as an alternative to feature detectors and hierarchies of classificatory units. These concepts are related to Perceptrons. Similarly, cell assemblies would find their technological analogue in a (non existing) Conceptron. ... It would be surprising if it turned out that the real brain makes use only of one or the other scheme. Most likely the two schemes are used in combination, with the hierarchical organization predominating at the sensory and motor periphery of the nervous system, and the cell assemblies in between. From this point of view the cerebral cortex would seem a good place for cell assemblies, and we have seen that it contains the necessary equipment" [125] p. 187*

Acknowledgements

The author is grateful to Karl Friston, Rosalyn Moran, Thomas Parr, Maxwell Ramstead, Vlad Krasnopolsky, Todd Hylton, Mark Latash for insightful comments and helpful discussions. Special thanks are due to Raj Malhotra of AFRL for supporting this and earlier work and for his help in evaluating ideas and steering the efforts towards their application. This material is based upon work supported by the Air Force Office of Scientific Research under award number FA9550-20-1-0013 and by the Air Force Research Laboratory under award number FA8650-19-C-1692. Any opinions, findings, and conclusions or recommendations expressed in this material are those of the author and do not necessarily reflect the views of the United States Air Force.

Author details

Yan M. Yufik
Virtual Structures Research, Inc., Potomac, MD, USA

*Address all correspondence to: imc.yufik@att.net

References

[1] Craik K. J. W. The Nature of Explanation. Cambridge University Press, Cambridge, UK. 1943.

[2] Rook L. L. Mental models: A robust definition. Faculty of Business - Papers (Archive). 1361 https://ro.uow.edu.au/buspapers/1361, 2013

[3] Doye, J. P. K., Wales, D. J. On potential energy surfaces and relaxation to the global minimum. J. Chem. Phys. 1996: 105, 8428-8445

[4] Moray N. Identifying mental models of complex human-machine systems. Int. J Industrial Ergonomics 1998: 22, 293-297.

[5] Moray N. Models of models of... mental models. In*:* Moray N. (ed). Ergonomics: Major Writings. Taylor and Francis, London, UK, 2004.p. 506-526.

[6] Rouse W. B., Morris N.N. On looking into the black box: prospects and limits in the search for mental models. Psychological Bulletin 1986: 100, 349-363.

[7] Johnson-Laird P.N. Mental models: Towards a cognitive science of language, inference, and consciousness. Cambridge University Press. N.Y. 1983

[8] Johnson- Laird P. N. Mental models and deduction. Trends in Cognitive Sciences 2001; 5, 10, 434-44

[9] Gentner D., Gentner. D. R. 1983. Flowing waters or teeming crowds: mental models of electricity. In: Gentner, D.A. Stevens A. (eds.) Mental Models. Lawrence Erlbaum, Hillsdale, New Jersey, USA, 1983; p. 99-130.

[10] Yufik Y.M. Virtual Associative Networks: A framework for cognitive modelling. In: Pribram K.H. (ed). Brain and Values. Lawrence Erlbaum Associates, New York, NY, 1998a: p. 109-177

[11] Yufik Y.M. Probabilistic Resource Allocation System with Self-Adaptive Capabilities, US Patent 5, 886, 219, 1998

[12] Yufik, Y.M. How the mind works: An exercise in pragmatism. In Proceedings. Int. Joint Conf. Neural Networks (IJCNN 02), Honolulu, HI, USA, 2002: p. 2265-2269.

[13] Friston K. J. Life as we know it. Journal Royal Society Interface 2013: 10, 20130475.

[14] Friston, K. J. The free-energy principle: A unified brain theory? Nature Review Neuroscience 2010; 11, 127-138

[15] Herculano–Housel S. The human brain in numbers: a linearly scaled-up primate brain. Frontiers Human Neuroscience. 2009; https://doi.org/10.3389/neuro.09.031.2009

[16] Schurmann T., Grassberg T. The predictability of letters in written English. arXiv:0710.4516 [physics.soc-ph] 2007.

[17] Chang M-C., Yang A. C-C., Stanley H.E., Peng C. K. Measuring information-base temperature and energy of literary texts. Physica A 2017; 468, p. 783-789

[18] Piaget J. 1975. The Development of Thought: Equilibration of Cognitive Structures. The Viking Press: New York, NY. 1975

[19] Freud, Z. The Joke and Its Relation to the Unconscious. Penguin Classics, 2003

[20] Bower T.G.R. Development in infancy. W.H. Freeman & Co. San Francisco, Ca. 1974

[21] Wright T. William Harvey: A life in circulation. Oxford University Press. 2013

[22] Aird W. C. Discovery of the cardiovascular system: From Galen to William Harvey. Journal of Thrombosis and Hemostasis 2011; 9, 118-129.

[23] Rovelli C. Reality is not what it seems. Riverhead Books. 2014

[24] Lehrer J. How we decide. Houghton Mifflin Harcourt. 2009

[25] Groot, A.D. Though and Choice in Chess. Basic Books Publishers: New York, NY. 1965

[26] Chen A.G., Benrimoh D., Parr T., Friston K. A Bayesian account of generalist and specialist formation under the active inference framework. Frontiers in Artificial Intelligence. https://doi.org/10.3389/frai.2020.00069; 2020

[27] Yufik Y. M. Understanding, consciousness and thermodynamics of cognition. Chaos Solitons Fractals. 2013; 55, 44-59.

[28] Yufik Y.M. Gnostron: A framework for human-like machine understanding. Proceedings. IEEE Symp. Computational Intelligence (SSCI), Bangalore, India 2019; 18-29.

[29] Yufik Y. M. The understanding capacity and information dynamics in the human brain. Entropy, 2019; 21, 308, p. 1-38.

[30] Yufik Y. M., Friston, K. J. Life and understanding: Origins of the understanding capacity in the self-organizing nervous system. Frontiers Systems Neuroscience. 2017; 10, 98.

[31] Cattell, R. B. Intelligence: Its Structure, Growth and Action. Elsevier, NY. 1978.

[32] Cattell R. B. 1971. Abilities: Their Structure, Growth, and Action. Houghton Mifflin, N.Y. 1971

[33] Cattell R. B. Theory of fluid and crystallized intelligence: A critical experiment. Journal Educational Psychology. 1963; 54, 1, 1-22.

[34] Harari, Y. N. Sapiens: A brief history of human kind. Harper Perennial. 2018.

[35] Chomsky, N. Biolinguistic explorations: design, development, evolution. International Journal Philosophical Studies. 2007: 15, 1-21.

[36] Hauser M.D., Chomsky N., Fitch, W.T. 2002. The faculty of language: what is it, who has it, and how did it evolve? Science, 2002; 298, 1569-1579.

[37] Berwick R. C., Chomsky, N. Why only us: language and evolution. The MIT Press. 2017.

[38] Caramelli 2008 Caramelli, D., Milani, L., Vai, S., Modi, A., Pecchioli, E., Girardi, M., Pilli, E., Lari, M., Lippi, B., Ronchitelli, A., Mallegni, F., Casoli, A., Bertorelle, B., Barbujani, G. 2008. A 28,000 years old Cro-Magnon mtDNA sequence differs from all potentially contaminating modern sequences. PLoS ONE 2008, 3(7): e2700.

[39] Hennenberg, D. 1988 Decrease of human skull size in the Holocene. Human Biology, 1988, 60(3), p. 395-405

[40] Calvin W.H. A brief history of the mind: From apes to intellect and beyond. Oxford University Press. NY. 2004

[41] Smaers J. B., Soligo C. Brain reorganization, not relative brain size, primarily characterizes anthropoid brain evolution. Proceedings Royal Society 2013; B 280: 20130269

[42] Deban S.M., Scales J.A., Bloom S.V., Easterling C.M., O'Donnell M.K., Jeffrey P., Olberding J.P. Evolution of a high-performance and functionally robust musculoskeletal system in

salamanders. Proceedings National Academy Sciences, 2020; 117 (19) p. 10445-10454

[43] Piaget J. The Grasp of Consciousness: Action and Concept in the Young Child. Taylor & Francis, NY. 1974

[44] Calvin W.H. The Cerebral Code. A Bradford Book. The MIT Press. 1996.

[45] Chomsky N. Biolinguistic explorations: design, development, evolution. International Journal Philosophical Studies. 2007; 15, p. 1-21.

[46] Piaget, J. Success and Understanding. Harvard University Press, Cambridge, MA. 1978

[47] Parr T., Friston, K. The anatomy of inference: Generative models and brain structures. Frontiers Computational Neuroscience. 2018; 12, 90

[48] Lear, J. Aristotle The desire to understand. Cambridge University Press. 1988.

[49] Rosen R. Life Itself. Columbia University Press. 1991.

[50] Haken, H. Synergetics: An Introduction. Nonequilibrium Phase Transitions and Self- Organization in Physics, Chemistry and Biology. Springer. 1996.

[51] Georgopoulos A.P. Lurito J.T., Petrides M., Schwartz A.B. Massey, J.T. Mental rotation of the neuronal population vector. Science, 1989; 243, 234-236.

[52] Georgopoulos A.P. Massey J.T. Cognitive spatial-motor processes 1. The making of movements at various angles from a stimulus direction. Experimental Brain Research. 1987; 65, p. 361-370

[53] Georgopoulos A.P., Taira, N., Lukashin, M. A. Cognitive neurophysiology of the motor cortex. Science. 1993, 260, 47-52.

[54] Papo D. Brain temperature: what it means and what it can do for (cognitive) neuroscientists, 2013: arXiv:1310.2906

[55] Koestler, A. The Act of Creation. Arkana, London, UK. 1964.

[56] James W. 1950. The Principles of Psychology. Dover Publications, NY, USA. 1950

[57] Fritz J. B., David S., Shamma S. Attention and dynamic, task-related receptive field plasticity in adult auditory cortex. In: Cohen Y.E., Popper A.N., Fay R.R. (ed) Neural Correlates of Auditory Cognition. Springer. 2013; p.251-290

[58] Fritz, J. B., Elhilali, M., & Shamma, S. A. Adaptive receptive field changes during detection of complex spectral targets. Journal of Neurophysiology. 2007, 98, p. 2337-2346

[59] Fritz, J. B., Elhilali, M., & Shamma, S. A. Active listening: Task-dependent plasticity of receptive fields in primary auditory cortex. Hearing Research, 2005; 206, 159-176.

[60] Fritz J. B., Shamma S. A., Elhilali M., & Klein, D. J. Rapid task-related plasticity of spectrotemporal receptive fields in primary auditory cortex. Nature Neuroscience. 2003; 6, p. 1216-1223.

[61] Atiani S., Elhilali M., David S. V., Fritz J. B., Shamma, S. A. (2009). Task difficulty and performance induce diverse adaptive patterns in gain and shape of primary auditory cortical receptive fields. Neuron. 2009; 61, p. 467-480.

[62] Duncan, J. An adaptive coding model of neural function in prefrontal

cortex. Nature Reviews Neuroscience, 2001; 2, 820-829.

[63] Stephen V. D., Fritz J.B., Shihab A. S. Proceedings National Academy Sciences, 2012; 109 (6) p. 2144-2149

[64] Christie S.T., Schrater P. Cognitive cost as dynamic allocation of energetic resources. Frontiers in Neuroscience, https://doi.org/10.3389/fnins.2015.00289, 2015

[65] Lieder F., Griffiths T.L. Resource--rational analysis: Understanding human cognition as the optimal use of limited computational resources. Behavioral Brain Sciences, 2019; 43, e1:1-60.

[66] Shaw, M.L., Shaw P. Optimal allocation of cognitive resources to spatial locations. Journal Experimental Psychology. 1977; 3(2), p.201-211.

[67] Dehaene S., Kerszberg M., Jean-Pierre Changeux J-P. A neuronal model of a global workspace in effortful cognitive tasks Proceedings National Academy Sciences 1998; 95 (24), p. 14529-14534

[68] Kouneiher F., Charon S., Koechlin E. Motivation and cognitive control in the human prefrontal cortex. Nature Neuroscience, 2009; 12 (7), p. 939-947.

[69] Kurzban R., Duckworth A., Kable, J.W., Myers, J. An opportunity cost model of subjective effort and task performance. Behavioral Brain Sciences, 2013. 36, p. 661-726

[70] Duncan J., Seltz R. J., Kolodny J., Bor D., Herzog H., Ahmed A., Newell F. N., Emslei H. A neural basis for general intelligence. Science, 2000; 289, 5478, p. 457-460

[71] Anderson M. L. Neural reuse: A fundamental organizational principle of the brain. Behavioral Brain Sciences, 2011; 33, p. 245-313.

[72] Bassett D. S., Greenfield D.L., Meyer-Lindenberg A., Weinberger, D. R., Moore, S. W., Bullmore, E.T. Efficient physical embedding of topologically complex information processing networks in brains and computer circuits. PLoS Computational Biology, 2010; 6, 4, e1000748

[73] Cherniak C., Mokhtarzada Z., Rodrigues-Esteban R., Changizi, K. Global optimization of cerebral cortex layout. Proceedings National Academy Sciences. 2004; 101, p. 1081-1086.

[74] Attwell D., Laughlin S. B. An energy budget for signaling in the grey matter of the brain. J Cereb Blood Flow Metab. 2001; 21, p. 1133-1145.

[75] Raichle M. E. , Mintun M. A. Brain work and brain imaging. Annual Reviews Neuroscience. 2006; 29:449-476.

[76] Rolfe et al, 1997; Rolfe, D. F., Brown GC. Cellular energy utilization and molecular origin of standard metabolic rate in mammals. Physiology Reviews, 1997; 77(3), 731-758.

[77] Shulman R. G., Rothman D. L., Behar K. L., Hyder, F. Energetic basis of brain activity: implications for neuroimaging. Trends Neurosci. 2004; 27, 489-495.

[78] Sengupta B., Stemmler M. B., Friston, K. J. Information and efficiency in the nervous system—A synthesis. PLoS Computational Biology, 2013; 9, 7: e1003157.

[79] Zhu X.-H., Qiao H., Du F., Xiong Q., Xiao L., Zhang X., Ugurbil K., Chen W. Quantitative imaging of energy expenditure in human brain, Neuroimage, 2012, 60 (4), p. 2107-2117.

[80] Tomasi, D., Wang, G.-J., Volkow, N. D. 2013. Energetic cost of brain functional connectivity. Proceedings National Academy Sciences, 2013; 110 (33), p. 13642-13647.

[81] Rae C., Scott R. B., Lee M., Simpson J. M., Hines N., Paul C., Anderson M., Karmiloff-Smith A., Styles, P., Radda, G.K. 2003. Brain bioenergetics and cognitive ability. Developmental Neuroscience, 2003, 25 (5) p. 324-331.

[82] Pepperell R. Consciousness as a physical process caused by the organization of energy in the brain. Frontiers in Psychology, 2019. https://ww.frontiersin.org/articles/10.3389/fpsyg.2018.02091/full

[83] Markman A.B., Otto, A.R. 2011. Cognitive systems optimize energy rather than information. Behavioral Brain Science, 2011; 34 (4), 207.

[84] Niven J. E., Laughlin S. B. Energy limitation as a selective pressure on the evolution of sensory systems. Journal Experimental Biology, 2008; 211, p. 1792-1804.

[85] Laughlin S.B., Attwell D. Neural energy consumption and representation of mental events. In: Shulman R.G., Rothman D. L.(eds.) Brain energetics and neuronal activity: Applications to fMRI and medicine. Wiley, 2004; p.11-124.

[86] Perin R., Berger T. K., Markram H. A synaptic organizing principle for cortical neuronal groups. PNAS 2011. 108 (13), p. 5419-5424

[87] Huang H.J., Kram R., Ahmed, A.A. Reduction of metabolic cost during motor learning of arm reaching dynamics. Journal of Neuroscience, 2012; 32960, p. 2182-2190.

[88] Sparrow W. A., Lay B. S., O'Dwyer N. J. Metabolic and attentional energy costs of interlimb coordination. Journal of Motor Behavior, 2007; 39 (4), p. 259-275

[89] Sparrow W. A., Newell K. 1998. Metabolic energy expenditure and the regulation of movement economy. Psychonomic Bulletin & Review. 1998; 5 (2), p. 173-196

[90] Sparrow W. A., Newell K. M. Energy expenditure and motor performance relationships in humans learning a motor task. Psychophysiology, 1994; 31, 338-346.

[91] Sparrow W. A., Irizarry-Lopez V. M. 1987. Mechanical efficiency and metabolic cost as measures of learning a novel gross-motor task. Journal Motor Behavior. 1987; 19, 240-264.

[92] Prilutsky, B. I. , Zatsiorsky, V. M. 2002. Optimization-based models of muscle coordination. Exercise Sport Science Reviews. 2002; 30, 32-38s

[93] O'Dwyer N. J., Neilson P. Metabolic energy expenditure and accuracy in movement: Relation to levels of muscle and cardiorespiratory activation and the sense of effort. In: Sparrow W. A. (ed.), Energetics of Human Activity. Human Kinetics, Champaign, 2002; p. 1-42

[94] Westbrook A., Braver T. S. 2015. Cognitive effort: A neuroeconomy approach. Cognitive, Affective Behavioral Neuroscience. 2015; 15, p. 395-415.

[95] Hebb, D.O. The organization of behavior. Wiley & Sons, N.Y. 1949.

[96] Edelman G. M., Gally J.A. 2013. Reentry: a key mechanism for integration of brain function. Frontiers in Integrative Neuroscience. 2013; 7, 63

[97] Edelman G. Neural Darwinism. The theory of neuronal group selection. Basic Books, NY. 1987.

[98] Edelman, G. Bright air, brilliant fire: On the matter of the mind. Basic Books, N.Y. 1992.

[99] Thoroughman K., Shadmehr R. Learning of action through adaptive

combination of motor primitives. Nature, 2000. 407, p. 742-747.

[100] Vyshedskiy, A. 2019. Neuroscience of imagination and implications for human evolution. Current Neurobiology 2019; 10 (2) p. 89-109.

[101] Lin L., Osan R. Tsien J.Z. Organizing principles of real-time memory encoding: Neural clique assemblies and universal neural codes. Trends Neuroscience. 2006; 29, 48-57

[102] Gelfand I. M, Latash M. L. On the problem of adequate language in movement science. Motor Control. 1998: 2, 306-313

[103] Gelfand, I. M., Latash M. L. On the problem of adequate language in biology. In: Latash M. L. (ed). Progress in Motor Control. vol. 2: Structure-Function Relations in Voluntary Movement. Human Kinetics, Urbana, IL, 2002. p. 209-228.

[104] Latash M. L. Biomechanics as a window into the neural control of movement. Journal Human Kinetics 2016; 52, 7-20.

[105] Latash M. L. Synergy. Oxford University Press, N. Y. 2008.

[106] Latash M. L. , Scholz J. P. , Schöner G. Toward a new theory of motor synergies. Motor Control. 2007; 11, 276-308

[107] Georgopoulos, A.P. Lurito, J.T., Petrides, M., Schwartz, A.B. Massey, J.T. 1989. Mental rotation of the neuronal population vector. Science, 1989: 243, p. 234-236.

[108] Georgopoulos A.P., Massey J.T. Cognitive spatial-motor processes 1. The making of movements at various angles from a stimulus direction. Experimental Brain Research. 1987: 65, p. 361-370.

[109] Georgopoulos A.P., Taira M., Lukashin, A. Cognitive neurophysiology of the motor cortex. Science 1993: 260, p. 47-52.

[110] Georgopoulos A.P., Kettner, R.E., Schwartz, A.B. Primate motor cortex and free arm movements to visual targets in three-dimensional space. II. Coding of the direction of movement by a neuronal population. Journal Neuroscience 8, 2928-2937.

[111] Latash M.L. Neurophysiological Basis of Movement. Human Kinetics. 2008.

[112] *Vaz A.P., Wittig Jr. J.H., Inati S.K., Zaghloul K.A.* Replay of cortical spiking sequences during human memory retrieval. Science, 2020: 367 (6482), p. 1131-1134

[113] Graybiel A.M. The basal ganglia and chunking of action repertoires. Neurobiology of Learning and Memory. 1998: 70, p. 119-136

[114] Jin X., Tecuapetla F., Costa R. M. 2014. Basal ganglia subcircuits distinctively encode the parsing and concatenation of action sequences, Nature Neuroscience. 2014. 17 (3), p. 423-430.

[115] Schmitt L., Wimmer R., Nakajima M., Happ M., Mofakham S., Halassa M.M. Thalamic amplification of cortical connectivity sustains attentional control. Nature 2017: 545, p. 219-223

[116] Miller R. Cortico-thalamic interplay and the security of operation of neural assemblies and temporal chains in the cerebral cortex. Biological Cybernetics 1996: 75, 263-275.

[117] Braitenberg V., Heck D., Sultan F. et al. The detection and generation of sequences as a key cerebellar function: Experiments and theory. Behavioral Brain Sciences 1997: 20 (2) p. 229-277.

[118] Bressler S. L., Kelso J.A. Coordination dynamics in cognitive

neuroscience. Frontiers in Neuroscience 2016, https://doi.org/10.3389/fnins.2016.00397

[119] Bressler S. L., Kelso J.A. Cortical coordination dynamics and cognition. Trends in Cognitive Neuroscience 2001:5(1) p. 26-36.

[120] Bressler S. L., Tognoli, E. Operational principles of neurocognitive networks. International Journal Psychophysiology. 2006: 60, 139-148.

[121] Kelso J.A.S., Dumas G., Tognoli E. Outline of a general theory of behavior and brain coordination. Neural Networks. 2013: 37, 120-131.,

[122] Edelman G. The remembered present: A biological theory of consciousness. Basic Books, NY. 1989.

[123] Edelman G. Bright air, brilliant fire: On the matter of the mind. Basic Books, N.Y. 1992.

[124] Edelman G., Changeaux, J-P. The Brain. Transaction Publishers. NY. 2001.

[125] Braitenberg, V. Cell assemblies in the cerebral cortex. In: Heim R., Palm G. (eds) Theoretical approaches to complex systems. Lecture Notes in Biomathematics, 21. Springer, Berlin, 1978: p. 171-188.

[126] Feldman, A.G., Goussev, V., Sangole, A., Levin, M.F. Threshold position control and the principle of minimal interaction in motor actions. Progress in Brain Research 2007: 165, p. 267-281.

[127] Feldman, A. G., Ostry, D.J., Levin, M. F., Gribble, P. L., Mitnitski, A. B. Recent tests of the equilibrium-point hypothesis (λ model). Motor Control 1998: 2, p. 189-205

[128] Feldman A.G., Levin M.F. The equilibrium-point hypothesis – past, present and future. In: Sternad D. (eds) Progress in Motor Control. Advances in Experimental Medicine and Biology, Springer, Boston, 2009. p. 699-726

[129] Doyle J., Ford D. Mental models concepts for system dynamics research. System Dynamics Review. 1998: 14 (1) p. 3-29

[130] Krivov S.V., Karplus M. Hidden complexity of free energy surfaces for peptide (protein) folding. Proceedings National Academy Sciences. 2004: 101 (41) p. 14766-14770

[131] Bryngelson J. D., Onuchic J. –N., Socci N. D., Wolynes P. G. Funnels, pathways and the energy landscape of protein folding: A Synthesis. Proteins 1995: 2 (3) p. 167-195

[132] Abeles M., Bergman H., Gat I., Meilijson I., Seidemann E., Tishby N., Vaadi E. Cortical activity flips among quasi-stationary states. Proceedings National Academy of Science. 1995: 92, p 8616-8620

[133] Miller E. K., Cohen J. D. 2001. An integrative theory of prefrontal function. Annual Reviews Neuroscience. 2001: 24, 167-202

[134] Tang E., Giusti G., Baum G.L., Gu S., , Pollock E., Kahn A.E., Roalf D.R. Moore T.M., Ruparel K., Gur R.C., Gur R.E., Satterthwaite T. D., Bassett D.S. Developmental increases in white matter network controllability support a growing diversity of brain dynamics. Nature Communications 2017: 18, 1252

[135] Ezaki T., Watanabe T., Ohzeki M., Masuda N. Energy landscape analysis of neuroimaging data. Philosophical Transactions Royal Society. 2017: A.37520160287

[136] Watanabe T., Hiroshe S., Wada H., Imal Y., Machida T., Shirouzu I., Konichi S., Miyashita Y., Masuda N., Energy landscapes of resting state brain

networks. Frontiers Neuroinformatics, 2014 https://doi.org/10.3389/fninf.2014.00012

[137] Gu, S., Cieslak, M., Baird, B., Muldoon, S.F., Grafton, S.T., Pasqualetti, F., Bassett, D.S. The energy landscape of neurophysiological activity implicit in brain network structure. Scientific Reports. 2018: 8, 2507, 1-15.

[138] Deco G., Jirsa V.K., McIntosh V.R. Resting brains never rest: Computational insights into potential cognitive architectures. Trends Neurocsience. 2013: 36 (5) p. 268-274

[139] Wei Y., de Lange S. C., Scholtens L. H., Watanabe K., Ardesch D. J., Jansen P. R., Savage J. E., Li L., Preuss T.M., James K., Rilling, J. K., Posthuma, D., van den Heuvel M.P. Genetic mapping and evolutionary analysis of human-expanded cognitive networks. Nature Communications, 2019: 10, 4839

[140] Raichle M. E. , Mintun M. A. Brain work and brain imaging. Annual Reviews Neuroscience. 2006: 29, p. 449-476.

[141] Seeley, W. W. The Salience Network: A neural system for perceiving and responding to homeostatic demands. Journal of Neuroscience, 2019: 39 (50) p. 9878-9882

[142] Nelson, S.M., Dosenbach, N.U.F., Cohen, A. L., Wheeler, M.E., Schlaggar, B.L., Petersen, S.E. Role of the anterior insula in task-level control and focal attention. Brain Structure Functions, 2010: 214, 5-6, p. 669-680.

[143] Smith, S.M., Fox, P.T., Miller, K. L., Glahn, D.C., Fox, P.M., Mackay, C.E., Filippini, N., Watkins, K.E., Toro, R., Angela R. Laird, A.R., Beckmann, C.F. Correspondence of the brain's functional architecture during activation and rest. PNAS 2009: 106, p. 31-42

[144] Klee, M.R., Pierau, F.-K., Faber, D.S. Temperature effects on resting potential and spike parameters of cat motoneurons. Experimental Brain Research 1974: 19, p. 478-492.

[145] Beggs, J. M., Plentz, D. Neuronal avalanches in neocortical circuits. Journal Neuroscience, 2003: 23 (35) p. 1167-11177.

[146] Goulden, N., Khusnulina, A., Davis, N.J., Bracewell R.M., , Bokde, A.L., McNulty, J.P., Mullins, P.G. The salience network is responsible for switching between the default mode network and the central executive network: Replication from DCM. Neuroimage, 2014: 99, p. 180-190.

[147] Amunts K., Schleicher, A., Zilles, K. Cytoarchitecture of the cerebral cortex. NeuroImage 2007: 37, p. 1061-1065

[148] Zilles, K., Amunts, K. 2015. Anatomical basis for functional specialization. In: Uludag, K., Ugurbil, K. & Berliner, L. (eds.). From nuclear spins to brain functions. Springer, 2015 p. 27-66.

[149] Hipolito I., Ramstead M., Convertino L., Bhat A., Friston K., Parr T. Markov Blankets in the Brain. 2020arXiv:2006.02741 **[q-bio.NC]**

[150] Buckner, R.L., Krienen, F.M. The evolution of distributed association networks in the human brain. Trends in Cognitive Sciences. 2013:17 (12), p.648-665.

[151] Laurent, G. What does 'understanding' mean?. Nature Neuroscience, 2000: **3,** 1211

[152] Hough A.R., Gluck K.A. The understanding problem in cognitive science. Advances in Cognitive Systems, 2019: 8, 13-32

[153] Waltz J.A., Knowlton B.J., Holoyak K.J., Boone K.B., Mishkin F.S., Santos M., Thomas C.R., Miller B.L. A system for relational reasoning in human prefrontal cortex. Psychological Science, 1999: 10 (2), p. 119-125.

[154] Krawczyk, D.C. The cognition and neuroscience of relational reasoning. Brain Research, 2012:1428, 13-23.

[155] Clement J. Creative model construction in scientists and students. Springer, The Netherlands 2008.

[156] Clement, J. J. The role of imagistic simulation in scientific thought experiments. Topics in Cognitive Science. 2009:1, p. 686-710

[157] Hegarty, M. Mechanical reasoning by mental simulation. Trends Cognitive Science. 2004: 8(6), p. 280-285.

[158] Kanai, R., Chang A., Yu, Y., de Abril, I. M., Biehl, M., Guttenberg, N. 2019. Information generation as a functional basis of consciousness. Neuroscience of Consciousness, 2019: 5, 1 niz016.

[159] Treisman, A. Focused attention in the perception and retrieval of multidimensional stimuli. Perception & Psychophysics, 1977: 22 (1) p. 1-11.

[160] Crick, F. Function of the thalamic reticular complex: The searchlight hypothesis. Proceedings National Academy Sciences. 1984: 81, 4586-4590.

[161] Rizzolatti, G., Arbib, M. 1998. Language within our grasp. Trends Neuroscience. 1998: 21 (5) p. 188-194.

[162] Friston, K. J., Parr, T., Yufik, Y., Sajid, N., Catherine J. Price, C. J., Holmes, E. Generative models, linguistic communication and active inference. Neuroscience and Biobehavioral Reviews. 2020: 118, p. 42-64.

[163] Pulvermuller, F. Words in the brain's language. Behavior and Brain Science. 1999: 22, p. 253-336.

[164] Pulvermuller, F. Hebb's concept of cell assemblies and the psychophysiology of word processing. Psychophysiology 1996: 33, p. 317-333

[165] Barsalou, L. W. Grounded cognition. Annual Reviews Psychology, 2008: 59, p. 617-645

[166] Boulenger, V., Hauk, O., Pulvermuller , F. Grasping ideas with the motor system: semantic somatotopy in idiom comprehension. Cerebral Cortex 2009: 19, p. 1905-1914

[167] Nelson, M. J., Karouib, I. E., Giberc, K., Yang, X., Cohen, L., Koopmanf, H., Cashc, S.C., Naccacheb, L., Haleg, J.T., Palliera, C., Dehaene, S. Neurophysiological dynamics of phrase-structure building during sentence processing Proceedings National Academy of Sciences, 2017: E3669–E3678

[168] Horwitz, B.; Rumsey, J.M.; Grady, C.L. The cerebral metabolic landscape in autism; intercorrelations of regional glucose utilization. Arch. Neurol. 1988, 45, 749-755.

[169] Just, M.A.; Cherkassky, V.L.; Keller, T.A.; Minshew, N.J. Cortical activation and synchronization during sentence comprehension in high-functioning autism: Evidence of underconnectivity. Brain 2004, 127,1811-1821.

[170] McAlonnan, G.M.; Cheung, V.; Cheung, C.; Suckling, J.; Lam, J.Y.; Tai, S.; Yip, L.; Murphy, D.G.M.; Chua, S.E. Mapping the brain in autism: A voxel-based MRI study of volumetric differences in autism. Brain 2005, 128, 268-276.

[171] Parsey, C. M., Schmitter-Edgecombe, M. Quantitative and

qualitative analyses of the clock drawing test in mild cognitive impairment and Alzheimer disease: Evaluation of a modified scoring system. Journal of Geriatric Psychiatry and Neurology. 2011; 24(2), p. 108-118.

[172] Smith, E., Morowitz, H. J. The Origin and Nature of Life on Earth. Cambridge University Press, U.K. 2016.

[173] Toyabe, S., Sagawa, T., Ueda, M. Muneyuki, E., Sano, M., 2010. Experimental demonstration of information-to-energy conversion and validation of the generalized Jarzynski equality. Nature Physics 2010: 6, p. 988-992

[174] Penrose, R. On understanding understanding. International Studies in the Philosophy of Science, 1997: 11 (1) p. 7-20

Chapter 5

The Neurofunctional Model of Consciousness: The Physiological Interconnectivity of Brain Networks

Umberto León-Domínguez

Abstract

The present chapter integrates neural networks' connectivity into a model that explores consciousness and volitional behavior from a neurofunctional perspective. The model poses a theoretical evidenced-based framework that organizes the brain journey of neural information flow from the ascending reticular activating system and non-specific thalamic nuclei, to cortical networks, such as the default mode network and the fronto-parietal network. These inter-connected brain networks can be divided within three hierarchical and inter-connected "functional neural loops": (1) the "brainstem-thalamic neural loop" for arousal, (2) the "thalamo-cortical neural loop" for neural information distribution throughout the brain, and (3) the "cortico-cortical neural loop" for transforming neural information into the contents of consciousness that the individual can perceive and manipulate voluntarily. These three neural loops act as a global functional neural system, and its disruption due to brain damage can cause a person to experience catastrophic outcomes, such as a coma, a vegetative state, a minimal conscious state, or other cognitive and behavioral impairments.

Keywords: consciousness, cortico-cortical system, thalamo-cortical system, brainstem, fronto-parietal network, default mode network

1. Introduction

Consciousness is a complex term to tackle objectively due to its broad epistemological spectrum. From a clinical view, consciousness has been neurophysiologically and behaviorally parameterized for its assessment [1, 2]. It is a central nervous process (reduccionism) that multiple neural long-range connections control (conexionism) and that is teleonomically goal directed. This neurofunctional point of view converges with theories about the emergence of new features in complex systems [3]. Various authors propose that high brain connectivity between distinct and distant neural groups is an elemental characteristic for the emergence of consciousness [3–5]. In this respect, consciousness is a neurophysiological phenomenon regulated by different brain networks that create *qualia*, the subjective experience of consciousness [6–11].

Consciousness should be interpreted as a physiological state of the central nervous system that changes over time and space. This functional mutability allows high-order cognitive functions to take place [6, 12, 13] to produce an overt and/or covert behavior that can be measured via direct observation or neuroimage [14–16]. All of these intermingled processes are supported via various brain networks that integrate endogenous and exogenous information with the intention of responding effectively to organic and psychological demands [6, 8, 11, 17, 18]. In this regard, acquired brain damage can impair the regular activity of brain networks, disorganizing cognition and behavior (mild, moderate, or severe brain damage), or even inhibiting the experience of consciousness (disorder of consciousness) [14, 19–21]. Therefore, from a clinical view, the structural and neurophysiological integrity of the neural substrate that underlies consciousness will determine the functional behavior of individuals [6, 22, 23]. Thus, consciousness can be described as a basal, dynamic, and transitive brain state that supports the high-order cognitive processing of information to produce suitable behaviors for environmental demands [24].

2. The neurofunctional model of consciousness

A huge number of theories seem to agree on many assumptions about consciousness, although they diverge regarding the descriptive approach. Some of them, such as the Global Neural Workspace Theory, focus on its neurophysiological components [11]. Meanwhile, others, such as the Global Workspace Theory, focus on its cognitive components [25]. In addition, the Integrated Information Theory focuses on its computational components [8, 26, 27]; the Temporo-Spatial Theory of Consciousness focuses on its inner space and time characteristics [6]; and the PFC-feedback System [28] focuses on its feedforward and feedback components. Crick and Koch introduced one of the first approaches to the study of consciousness [9]. Their approach posits that the experience of consciousness will be determined based on the long-range connectivity between the front and back parts of the brain. All of these authors and theories have shed light on the phenomena of consciousness and have probably contributed to the very first theoretical foundations for the study of consciousness objectively:

- Consciousness depends on bioelectrical and biochemical brain activity.
- Some neurophysiological processes are required to experience consciousness as awareness (i.e., the object or event has to trigger a P300 wave on the cortex).
- These neurophysiological processes are regulated via various neural groups that process information in a rapid, automatic, and stereotypical manner (back brain), as well as via other neural groups that process information in a slow and voluntary manner (front brain).
- Consciousness needs long-range connectivity between distinct and distant brain areas.
- These long-range connections (probably in beta bands) assemble distinct and distant neural groups into extended neural networks that regulate various physiological and phenomenological dimensions that are necessary for the experience of consciousness.

One of the main neural models that are emerging currently about neural processing is the "predictive coding model" [29, 30]. This model posits that neural processing occurs within feedforward and feedback loops between upper and lower brain structures and slices. Lower structures/slices send predictions to upper structures and these structures send back error predictions to adjust neural processes to make the ongoing behavior efficient [29–33]. Llinás has already suggested that consciousness could be more related to a close-loop neural network than to the emergent consequence of a sensory input [34]. In this sense, a functional and preserved consciousness could depend on the predictive codification between inferior (brainstem and thalamus) and superior brain structures (cortex), where the prefrontal cortex (PFC) receives "end-of-the-line" bottom-up predictions and sends top-down error predictions to the thalamus to adjust new top-down projections [24, 35–40].

Despite all of the theories and experimental evidence about the neural networks involved in consciousness, no global theoretical framework exists to describe how these neural networks operate to produce and maintain consciousness. The present chapter will introduce a neurofunctional model that organizes the interaction and functioning of the neural networks into three neurofunctional loops: (1) the Brainstem-Thalamic neural loop (B-T neural loop), (2) the Thalamo-Cortical neural loop (T-C neural loop), and (3) the Cortico-Cortical neural loop (C-C Neural Loop). Each of these loops are formed via differentiated and semi-independent neural structures that are involved in specific aspects of the phenomenological consciousness.

2.1 B-T neural loop

The brainstem plays a key role in the regulation of consciousness due to the control that it exerts to the Ascending Reticular Activating System (ARAS) and therefore to wakefulness (wakefulness and awareness are the two clinical dimensions typically related to consciousness) [41, 42]. The ARAS is composed of myriad brainstem nuclei (dorsal raphe locus coeruleus, median raphe, pedunculopontine, and parabrachial nuclei), with connections to the thalamus, hypothalamus, and basal forebrain [42–48], and even with the prefrontal areas [49] and the precuneus (Pcu) [50]. The lower dorsal ARAS connects the pontine reticular formation to the intralaminar thalamic nuclei (ILN), the lower ventral ARAS connects the pontine reticular formation to the hypothalamus, and the upper ARAS connects the intralaminar thalamic nuclei to the cerebral cortex [51–54]. Whereas hypothalamic-basal forebrain pathways regulate sleep-wakefulness cycles [48, 55, 56], the ILN, as part of the non-specific thalamic nuclei, can block thalamocortical rhythms and therefore the emergence of arousal and awareness [22, 57–60]. Baars [18] called this circuit the Extended Reticular-Thalamic Activating System, which he considered to be the principal neural assembly in the experience of consciousness.

2.2 T-C neural loop

A significant amount of evidence points out that reciprocal interactions between the thalamus and cortex are a fundamental component of the proper functioning of the thalamo-cortical system [61], which is related to consciousness [62]. This thalamo-cortico-thalamic connectivity starts to develop in the late prenatal and early postnatal stages [61, 63, 64], and the efficient deployment of these developmental processes will determine the functional state of the thalamo-cortical system in the adult stage [65]. The thalamus has been proposed as the main neural structure of the thalamo-cortical system, as it operates as a regulator of cortical functional connectivity, whereby it is involved in the ongoing cognitive processes [66–70]. The thalamus can be divided into three nuclear groups: first-order thalamic relay nuclei, higher-order thalamic relay nuclei, or non-specific thalamic nuclei. First-order thalamic nuclei send afferent projections to the primary sensory cortical areas, whereas higher-order nuclei receive projections from the primary sensory cortical areas and send these projections back to the higher visual cortical areas forming the cortico-thalamo-cortico circuits. Finally, nonspecific thalamic nuclei are those that receive projections from the ARAS and send diffuse projections throughout the brain [71–73]. The nonspecific thalamic nuclei are composed of three main nuclear groups: the thalamic reticular nucleus (TRN), the ILN, and the midline thalamic nuclei (MTN). The TRN-ILN-MTN thalamic axis has been related to consciousness [22, 62, 74] with strong implications in the distribution of neural information throughout the brain [24].

The functional extent of each nonspecific thalamic nuclei is related to the control and regulation of a specific cognitive domain [24] . The TRN is one of the main neural nodes that regulates the activity of the thalamus and therefore the activity of the entire thalamo-cortical system [75–77]. The TRN receives afferent glutamatergic projections from the entire brain, and in turn, it sends only efferent GABAergic projections to the thalamus, thus regulating thalamo-cortical and cortico-cortical activity [28, 78, 79]. On a morphological level, the TRN is divided into sensory and motor regions [80]. Whereas the sensory region modulates attentional processes via connections with the prefrontal cortex [38], the motor region is involved in limbic and motor processes due to high connectivity with the ILN-NMT, the ventrolateral, and the anterior thalamic nuclei [81–85]. Various authors have referred to the involvement of the TRN in the attentional processes as the "attention spotlight" and "attentional door" that regulate the flow of information between the thalamus and the cortex [35, 86, 87]. The capacity to control neural information throughout the brain is due to the inhibition that it exerts to the thalamic nuclei [37, 76, 86]. This inhibition mechanism underlying the "attention spotlight" selects the information needed to face psychological and physiological demands while suppressing those that are not relevant. Some authors suggest that the TRN is involved in the content of consciousness by controlling selective attentional processes and the thalamus activity [28, 86]. According to Crick [35], the short-term synaptic plasticity of the TRN could influence first-order thalamic relay nuclei in the formation of temporal connections between brain areas related to the content of consciousness [35]. Hence, this capacity to modulate the content of consciousness could be mediated by the control of attentional processes [88–90].

On the other hand, the functions of the ILN and the MTN are functionally differentiated, but their activity are highly dependent [91–95]. Regarding consciousness, both nuclei (due to its multiple connections with the ARAS) activate the excitability of the cerebral cortex to maintain vigilance and arousal [42, 58–60, 76, 91]. For instance, the ILN send and receive projections from the prefrontal, motor, and parietal cortices. Meanwhile, the MTN is connected to the medial prefrontal cortex (mPFC) and the hippocampus (HPC). These diffuse connections spread to the cortex, thus allowing the synchronization of brain activity through the adjustment of the brain waves' phases. Thus, distinct and distant neural groups assemble into cortico-cortical networks to facilitate the flow of neural information [91]. In addition, The ILN and MTN are also involved in the regulation of the striatal-thalamocortical circuits [96] due to the multiple efferent inhibitory connections that receive from the TRN, the basal ganglia, and the reticular formation of the ARAS [97–99]. These connections with the striatum, the brainstem, and the cortex highlight the relevance of the ILN and the MTN in the motor, somatic, and visceral functions, which are essential for controlling arousal, perception, and even emotion expression [100].

Specifically, the ILN have been associated with the regulation of cortical activity and the restoration of consciousness [22, 68, 101, 102]. The anterior region of the ILN react to motor inputs [103, 104], whereas the posterior region organizes motor, limbic, and associative information [60, 97, 105, 106]. Projections to limbic structures and sensori-motor areas suggest the relevance of the integration of the affective and motor functions that underly propositional behaviors [107]. In addition, they are involved in tasks that require the focalization of attention and the selection of actions for unexpected events [108, 109]. Kinomura and colleagues pointed out that arousal and attention require the simultaneous activation of the reticular formation of the midbrain and the ILN [110]. This evidence places the ILN as the basic neural nodes for the integration of brain functions, such as arousal, attention, and motor control, to trigger high-level cognitive performance [86, 104, 110–113]. This functional characteristic of the ILN in the regulation of the arousal has been employed for deep brain stimulation in cases of minimally conscious state. Schiff [22, 114] showed that stimulating the ILN in minimally conscious state patients could improve their motor behavior, but without showing any sign of "real" consciousness [22, 114, 115]. Therefore, although the ILN seems to be involved in consciousness, it cannot produce a constant and fluent stream of consciousness by itself.

Finally, the MTN have been reported as the main "gateway" of information to the HPC and the limbic system, with a high dependence on the individual's arousal levels [116–119]. Concretely, the nucleus reuniens and rhomboid of the MTN jointly with the mPFC and the HPC form a specialized neural circuit that contribute to learning and to the cognitive flexibility [120], probably due to its relationship with the working memory [116, 117]. This circuit constituted by the MTN-HPC-mPFC could be modified via the functional state of the TRN [121] and also affect the content of consciousness [122]. Other authors propose that the circuit formed via the orbital and mPFC, the amygdala, the hypothalamus, and the MTN could also be involved in the visceral and emotional control of human behavior [123–128]. The MTN directly influences the arousal and attentional processes through its involvement in emotional regulation [129]. Thence, it is implicated in the emotional adjustment of behavior in a continuously changing environment [130]. According to these authors, the MTN could mediate the selection of the most suitable behavior depending on the emotional tone inputs received in a specific moment [118, 130]. This evidence places the MTN as a remarkable interface between the diverse structures of the limbic system to integrate memory, emotion, and cognition [100, 119, 129, 131].

All of this evidence points out that the TRN-ILN-MTX thalamic axis and its connections throughout the brain are essential components for being conscious and aware of our surroundings due to the axis's capacity to place the T-C neural loop in an optimal functional state [24, 35]. In this sense, it is important to distinguish between "be aware" and the "formation of consciousness." Being aware of something means that our cognitive systems are prepared to receive and manipulate the content of consciousness, but the formation of the content of consciousness depends on other neural processes. The content of consciousness is formed mainly in the posterior cortex [132, 133] through cortico-thalamo-cortico circuits, which facilitate connections among various sensory cortical areas in the "content-specific Neural Correlates of Consciousness (NCC)" [70, 133–136]. Regardless of the content-specific NCC, when it comes to accessing consciousness, some neurophysiological requirements, such as a late P300 wave, are needed to ignite a global brain activation that will trigger awareness [137]. The conscious perception of the content of consciousness is the end of the concatenation of neurophysiological events that propagate from the back to the front cortex [6, 138]. It would be like a competition among various neural coalitions to access consciousness, and once a winning coalition exists (the first to break neurophysiological requirements), a specific representation or the content of consciousness can be perceived as generating a genuine experience of consciousness [137]. Afterward, this content of consciousness is controlled by high-order cognitive functions and is incorporated into plans, desires, and/or thoughts [6, 139].

2.3 C-C neural loop

Once the content of consciousness is created in the back brain [132, 133], various cortico-cortical networks consciously manipulate the information [140]. One of the main cortico-cortical networks, which is broadly documented, is the Default Mode Network (DMN) [141–144]. This network is formed by the anterior and posterior cingulate cortex, the mPFC, the orbital PFC, the medial temporal lobe (parahippocampal cortex and HPC), the retrosplenial cortex, and the inferior parietal lobe [145] . The DMN is a rest neural network, whose activity is maximum when the subject is awake and the cognitive demand is low (low-level processing of exogenous information) [146]. Moreover, the DMN is characterized by a high metabolism during rest states [147–150], a progressive deactivation when more cognitive resources are needed to process information [147], and a high connectivity with other cortico-cortical networks to exchange information [140, 143, 151]. Traditionally, the DMN has been related to internal processes, such as self-reference thoughts and mind-wandering [152–154], although some studies currently link its activity to extrinsic processes, such as certain attentional processes [155] and the recall of memories [156–159]. Recently, it has been posed that the DMN could also be involved in the integration of spatial, self-reference, and temporal information, thus generating episodic memories [160]. These authors suggest that, henceforth, the DMN is mostly activated in all of the cognitive processes [160].

One of the key points for understanding the role of the DMN in consciousness is to conceive it as a cognitive system that modulate cortico-cortical activity through its mediation in the transfer of information from resting states or task-negative networks to cognitively active states or task-positive networks [140, 147, 156, 161–164]. When a subject is resting (with the low-level processing of exogenous information), the DMN controls cortical activity with the posterior cingulate cortex (PCC) and the precuneus (Pcu) as their main neural nodes. However, as long as elaborated processing is required and the load of the working memory increases, the physiological burden of the DMN decreases in favor of task-positive networks: the fronto-parietal central executive network (FPN), the dorsal attention network (DAN), and the salience network (SN). The FPN includes the dorsolateral PFC, the mPFC, the anterior insula (aINS), the Pcu, and the interior parietal lobe [140, 165–167]. On the other hand, the DAN is formed by the frontal eye field and the intraparietal sulcus [168], and the SN by the aINS, the dorsal anterior cingulate cortex, the amygdala, the ventral striatum, and the ventral tegmental area of the mesencephalon [169]. All of these networks share overlapping regions whereby they can exchange neural information depending on the ongoing cognitive activity [147, 149, 150, 170–173] . The outcome of the continuous interactions among the cortico-cortical networks will define the functional conscious state of the individual [163].

The FPN, DAN, and SN play a key role in conscious behavior due to its capacity to operate jointly and synchronically in a highly coordinated and temporally accurate manner [140, 165, 174]. For instance, the DAN has been related to focalized attention and working memory, whereas the SN has been related to social communication, social behavior, and self-consciousness [171, 175–178] . When all of these task-positive networks are operating, the DMN needs to deactivate [179–181] to facilitate the transition from low-energy cognitive states to high-energy cognitive states [147]. In these high-energy cognitive states, the mPFC takes control of the global brain activity at the expense of the PCC and the Pcu [170, 182]. Therefore, the alteration of structural and functional connectivity "within and between cortico-cortical networks" could cause the individual to experience a broad spectrum of neuropsychiatric and neurocognitive disorders [162, 163, 180, 183, 184].

The FPN and SN, especially in the prefrontal regions, regulate the cognitive processes involved in the achievement of conscious goals through the regulation of the physiological *equilibrium* between the DMN and the rest of the cortico-cortical networks (cognitive control) [140, 165–167, 185, 186]. Some studies point out that the mPFC and aINS regulate physiological *equilibrium* among brain networks [178, 187]. For instance, Crone and colleagues compared the activation/deactivation of the DMN in vegetative states (currently known as "unresponsive wakefulness state"), minimally conscious states, and individuals with preserved and functional consciousness (control subjects) [182]. They suggested that although the deactivation of the DMN was normal in control subjects, the same deactivation was significantly diminished in overlapped areas between the DMN and the FPN in a minimally conscious state, and it was absent in unresponsive wakefulness state patients. In other words, the cohesive and functional integrity between the DMN and the task-positive networks is a crucial factor in the transition between rest states (those with a low cognitive burden) to high-demand cognitive states (those with a high cognitive burden) [147]. Our team conducted an investigation whereby we compared cortical connectivity between minimally conscious states and severe neurocognitive disorders [4]. Our results revealed how the degree of connectivity between the anterior and the posterior cortex in the beta band was essential for maintaining a preserved consciousness. In this investigation, patients with minimally conscious states showed a low connectivity between the posterior and the anterior cortex, which could explain why their consciousness fluctuates over time [4]. In contrast, subjects with preserved consciousness showed a high connectivity between the anterior and the posterior cortex, whereby they can operate continuously without the absence of consciousness [4]. In this sense, in a case study, an unresponsive conscious patient emerged to a minimally conscious state when connectivity between the anterior and the posterior cortex increased [188]. Thus, the integration of the posterior and the anterior cortex into long-distance cortico-cortical networks is one of the principal prerequisites for maintaining functional consciousness [9, 182, 189, 190].

3. Assumptions for the neuroFunctional Model of Consciousness (nFMC)

1. The nFMC is a theoretical and referential framework from which the study of consciousness can be tackled in all of its operative dimensions: neurophysiological, clinical, neuropharmacological, and phenomenological.

2. Consciousness is a global neural process that keeps the individual in an optimal and continuous functional state, thus allowing qualia and high-order processes to take place to drive behavior.

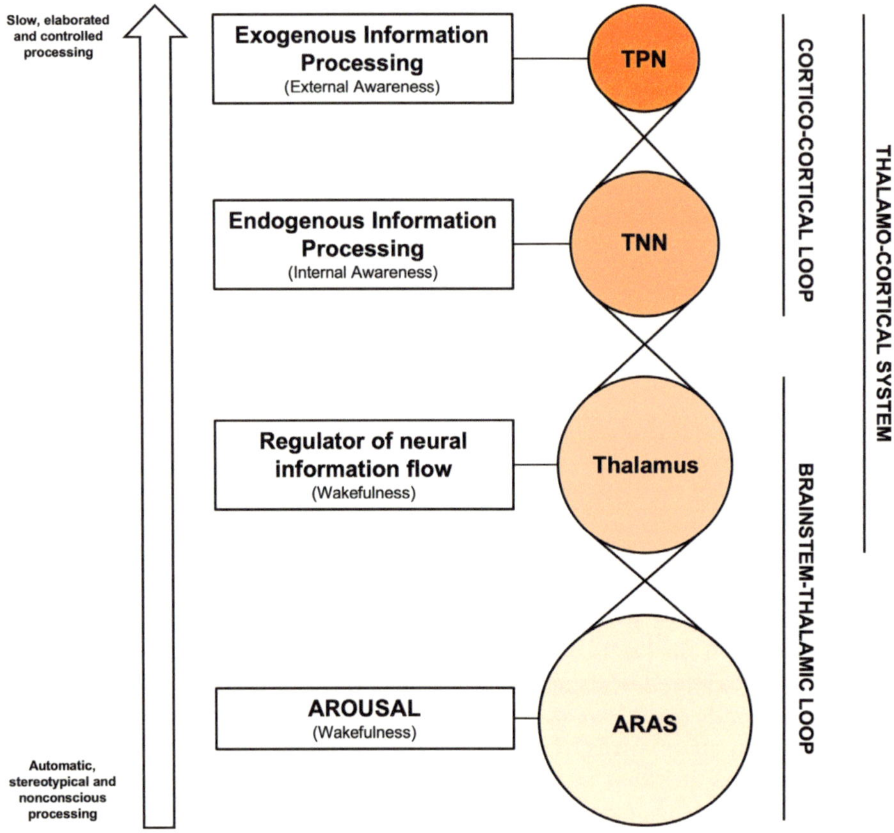

Figure 1.
Consciousness is the phenomenological quality of human existence that arises from a hierarchical, parallel, and serial activation of long-distance brain networks [7], which operate as neural loops that "inform" upper and lower levels about their own operations [29, 30]. These loops receive input from lower levels (which contains new information/predictions) and input from upper levels (error predictions). The loop will integrate all of this new information, updating its own functional state and, consequently, also the functional state of the rest of the loops and the brain [29–32, 191]. ***ARAS:*** *Ascending reticular activating system;* ***TNN:*** *Task-negative networks;* ***TPN:*** *Task-positive networks.*

3. The nFMC divides global neural activity into three large systems, or functional loops, that are morphologically differentiated (although they share overlapped areas) and have semi-independent neurophysiological processes: the B-T neural loop, T-C neural loop, and C-C neural loop (see **Figure 1**).

4. Cognitive, behavioral, and emotional expression due to brain damage will depend on the location and extension of the lesion within the neural loop, thus leading to clinical outcomes that they may vary from a mild cognitive impairment to a disorder of consciousness, such as a coma, minimally conscious state, or unresponsive wakefulness state.

5. Each neural loop is activated hierarchically and sequentially by its preceding level, thus extending a representation of the neural processes that took place in the lower level, as well as integrating and transforming this neural representation into new information.

6. The nFMC is in accordance with predictive coding models that present brain activity as a system in which lower brain structures project predictions/signals

via bottom–up processing, and where higher cortical areas send prediction errors back via top-down processes.

7. Neural processes (both automatic and controlled) related to consciousness (such as P300, brain rhythms, and neurotransmitter discharges) can be localized within either of the neural loops or in their reciprocal interactions.

8. The nFMC is complementary and comprises several assumptions considered in previous theories and investigations of consciousness:

    - Consciousness can be deemed a Global Neural Workspace in which distinct neural networks compete to access consciousness [11, 25, 192].

    - Consciousness is the result of functional units or complexes that integrate information and that are activated or deactivated depending on the ongoing sensorial/visceral necessities [8, 26, 27].

    - Consciousness is a neurophysiological continuum commanded by inner spatio-temporal brain laws [6].

9. Regarding the neural mechanisms or processes involved in the formation of the content of consciousness, the nFMC aligns with models and evidence that posit that the contents of consciousness are formed in the back brain via cortico-thalamo-cortical connections [70, 132–136]. In addition, the nFMC recognizes that PFC top-down connections could modulate the selection and even the formation of the content of consciousness [28].

4. Conclusion

Human behavior has to be understood as a global brain activity dominated by complex and hierarchical neural processes that cannot be divided and explained by isolated functional units. Consciousness is the "operating system" running underneath the "interface" of overt and covert human behavior, and it is dominated by the interactions of various neural levels composed of differentiated and semi-independent neural networks. Thence, the nFMC gathers reliable knowledge generated in the study on neural correlates of consciousness, providing a novel theoretical and referential framework that will help clinicians, researchers, and even students to localize the neural processes of interest within a global brain activity model. A further proposal should extend the structures and connectivity involved within and between each neural loop introduced in the nFMC.

Conflict of interest

The authors have no conflict of interest to declare.

Author details

Umberto León-Domínguez
Human Cognition and Brain Research Lab, School of Psychology, University of Monterrey, San Pedro Garza García, Mexico

*Address all correspondence to: umberto.leon@udem.edu

References

[1] Wolff A, Di Giovanni DA, Gómez-Pilar J, et al. The temporal signature of self: Temporal measures of resting-state EEG predict self-consciousness. *Hum Brain Mapp*. Epub ahead of print 4 October 2018. DOI: 10.1002/hbm.24412.

[2] Teasdale G, Jennett B. Assessment of coma and impaired consciousness. A practical scale. *Lancet (London, England)* 1974; 2: 81-4.

[3] Godwin D, Barry RL, Marois R. Breakdown of the brain's functional network modularity with awareness. *Proc Natl Acad Sci U S A* 2015; 112: 3799-804.

[4] Leon-Carrion J, Leon-Dominguez U, Pollonini L, et al. Synchronization between the anterior and posterior cortex determines consciousness level in patients with traumatic brain injury (TBI). *Brain Res* 2012; 1476: 22-30.

[5] Leon-Dominguez U, Izzetoglu M, Leon-Carrion J, et al. Molecular concentration of deoxyHb in human prefrontal cortex predicts the emergence and suppression of consciousness. *Neuroimage* 2014; 85 Pt 1: 616-25.

[6] Northoff G, Huang Z. How do the brain's time and space mediate consciousness and its different dimensions? Temporo-spatial theory of consciousness (TTC). *Neurosci Biobehav Rev* 2017; 80: 630-645.

[7] John ER, Prichep LS. The anesthetic cascade: a theory of how anesthesia suppresses consciousness. *Anesthesiology* 2005; 102: 447-71.

[8] Tononi G. An information integration theory of consciousness. *BMC Neurosci* 2004; 5: 42.

[9] Crick F, Koch C. Are we aware of neural activity in primary visual cortex? *Nature* 1995; 375: 121-123.

[10] Edelman GM, Gally JA, Baars BJ. Biology of Consciousness. *Front Psychol* 2011; 2: 4.

[11] Dehaene S, Kerszberg M, Changeux JP. A neuronal model of a global workspace in effortful cognitive tasks. *Proc Natl Acad Sci U S A* 1998; 95: 14529-34.

[12] Northoff G. What the brain's intrinsic activity can tell us about consciousness? A tri-dimensional view. *Neurosci Biobehav Rev* 2013; 37: 726-38.

[13] Singer W. Consciousness and the binding problem. *Ann N Y Acad Sci* 2001; 929: 123-46.

[14] Giacino JT, Ashwal S, Childs N, et al. The minimally conscious state: definition and diagnostic criteria. *Neurology* 2002; 58: 349-53.

[15] Owen AM, Coleman MR, Boly M, et al. Detecting Awareness in the Vegetative State. *Science (80-)* 2006; 313: 1402-1402.

[16] Bai Y, Xia X, Li X. A Review of Resting-State Electroencephalography Analysis in Disorders of Consciousness. *Front Neurol* 2017; 8: 471.

[17] Crick F, Koch C. A framework for consciousness. *Nat Neurosci* 2003; 6: 119-126.

[18] Baars BJ. *A cognitive theory of consciousness*. Cambridge University Press, 1993.

[19] Laureys S, Faymonville ME, Luxen A, et al. Restoration of thalamocortical connectivity after recovery from persistent vegetative state. *Lancet (London, England)* 2000; 355: 1790-1.

[20] León-Carrión J. Dementia Due to Head Trauma: An obscure name for a clear neurocognitive syndrome. *NeuroRehabilitation* 2002; 17: 115-22.

[21] Riddoch MJ, Humphreys GW. Visual agnosia. *Neurol Clin* 2003; 21: 501-20.

[22] Schiff ND. Central thalamic contributions to arousal regulation and neurological disorders of consciousness. *Ann N Y Acad Sci* 2008; 1129: 105-18.

[23] Fernández-Espejo D, Bekinschtein T, Monti MM, et al. Diffusion weighted imaging distinguishes the vegetative state from the minimally conscious state. *Neuroimage* 2011; 54: 103-12.

[24] León-Domínguez U, Vela-Bueno A, Froufé-Torres M, et al. A chronometric functional sub-network in the thalamo-cortical system regulates the flow of neural information necessary for conscious cognitive processes. *Neuropsychologia* 2013; 51: 1336-1349.

[25] Baars BJ. Global workspace theory of consciousness: toward a cognitive neuroscience of human experience. *Prog Brain Res* 2005; 150: 45-53.

[26] Tononi G, Edelman GM. Consciousness and complexity. *Science* 1998; 282: 1846-51.

[27] Tononi G, Boly M, Massimini M, et al. Integrated information theory: from consciousness to its physical substrate. *Nat Rev Neurosci* 2016; 17: 450-61.

[28] León-Domínguez U, León-Carrión J. Prefrontal neural dynamics in consciousness. *Neuropsychologia*; 131. Epub ahead of print 2019. DOI: 10.1016/j.neuropsychologia.2019.05.018.

[29] Friston K. The free-energy principle: a unified brain theory? *Nat Rev Neurosci* 2010; 11: 127-138.

[30] Friston K. The free-energy principle: a rough guide to the brain? *Trends Cogn Sci* 2009; 13: 293-301.

[31] Rao RPN, Ballard DH. Predictive coding in the visual cortex: a functional interpretation of some extra-classical receptive-field effects. *Nat Neurosci* 1999; 2: 79-87.

[32] Lee TS, Mumford D. Hierarchical Bayesian inference in the visual cortex. *J Opt Soc Am A Opt Image Sci Vis* 2003; 20: 1434-48.

[33] Kellermann T, Scholle R, Schneider F, et al. Decreasing predictability of visual motion enhances feed-forward processing in visual cortex when stimuli are behaviorally relevant. *Brain Struct Funct* 2017; 222: 849-866.

[34] Llinás RR, Paré D. Of dreaming and wakefulness. *Neuroscience* 1991; 44: 521-35.

[35] Crick F. Function of the thalamic reticular complex: the searchlight hypothesis. *Proc Natl Acad Sci U S A* 1984; 81: 4586-90.

[36] Barbas H, García-Cabezas MÁ. How the prefrontal executive got its stripes. *Curr Opin Neurobiol* 2016; 40: 125-134.

[37] Zikopoulos B, Barbas H. Pathways for emotions and attention converge on the thalamic reticular nucleus in primates. *J Neurosci* 2012; 32: 5338-50.

[38] Zikopoulos B, Barbas H. Prefrontal projections to the thalamic reticular nucleus form a unique circuit for attentional mechanisms. *J Neurosci* 2006; 26: 7348-61.

[39] Chanes L, Barrett LF. Redefining the Role of Limbic Areas in Cortical Processing. *Trends Cogn Sci* 2016; 20: 96-106.

[40] Alexander WH, Brown JW. Frontal cortex function as derived from hierarchical predictive coding. *Sci Rep* 2018; 8: 3843.

[41] Laureys S. The neural correlate of (un)awareness: lessons from the vegetative state. *Trends Cogn Sci* 2005; 9: 556-9.

[42] Moruzzi G, Magoun HW. Brain stem reticular formation and activation of the EEG. *Electroencephalogr Clin Neurophysiol* 1949; 1: 455-73.

[43] Långsjö JW, Alkire MT, Kaskinoro K, et al. Returning from oblivion: imaging the neural core of consciousness. *J Neurosci* 2012; 32: 4935-43.

[44] Jones BE. Arousal systems. *Front Biosci* 2003; 8: s438-51.

[45] Kolmac CI, Mitrofanis J. Patterns of brainstem projection to the thalamic reticular nucleus. *J Comp Neurol* 1998; 396: 531-43.

[46] Fuller PM, Fuller P, Sherman D, et al. Reassessment of the structural basis of the ascending arousal system. *J Comp Neurol* 2011; 519: 933-56.

[47] Parvizi J, Damasio AR. Neuroanatomical correlates of brainstem coma. *Brain* 2003; 126: 1524-1536.

[48] Jang SH, Kwon HG. The Neural Tract Between the Hypothalamus and Basal Forebrain in the Ascending Reticular Activating System: A Diffusion Tensor Tractography Study. *Curr Med Imaging Rev* 2019; 15: 369-372.

[49] SH J, HG K. The direct pathway from the brainstem reticular formation to the cerebral cortex in the ascending reticular activating system: A diffusion tensor imaging study. *Neurosci Lett*; 606. Epub ahead of print 2015. DOI: 10.1016/J.NEULET.2015.09.004.

[50] Silva S, Alacoque X, Fourcade O, et al. Wakefulness and loss of awareness: Brain and brainstem interaction in the vegetative state. *Neurology* 2010; 74: 313-320.

[51] Jang SH, Kwon HG. The ascending reticular activating system from pontine reticular formation to the hypothalamus in the human brain: a diffusion tensor imaging study. *Neurosci Lett* 2015; 590: 58-61.

[52] Yeo SS, Chang PH, Jang SH. The ascending reticular activating system from pontine reticular formation to the thalamus in the human brain. *Front Hum Neurosci* 2013; 7: 416.

[53] Berry DJ, Ohara PT, Jeffery G, et al. Are there connections between the thalamic reticular nucleus and the brainstem reticular formation? *J Comp Neurol* 1986; 243: 347-62.

[54] Jang SH, Kwon YH. Neuroimaging characterization of recovery of impaired consciousness in patients with disorders of consciousness. *Neural Regen Res* 2019; 14: 1202-1207.

[55] Kostin A, Siegel JM, Alam MN. Lack of Hypocretin Attenuates Behavioral Changes Produced by Glutamatergic Activation of the Perifornical-Lateral Hypothalamic Area. *Sleep* 2014; 37: 1011-1020.

[56] Naganuma F, Bandaru SS, Absi G, et al. Melanin-concentrating hormone neurons contribute to dysregulation of rapid eye movement sleep in narcolepsy. *Neurobiol Dis* 2018; 120: 12-20.

[57] McCormick DA. Cholinergic and noradrenergic modulation of thalamocortical processing. *Trends Neurosci* 1989; 12: 215-21.

[58] Lavoie B, Parent A. Serotoninergic innervation of the thalamus in the primate: An immunohistochemical study. *J Comp Neurol* 1991; 312: 1-18.

[59] Oke AF, Carver LA, Gouvion CM, et al. Three-dimensional mapping of norepinephrine and serotonin in human thalamus. *Brain Res* 1997; 763: 69-78.

[60] Krout KE, Belzer RE, Loewy AD. Brainstem projections to midline and intralaminar thalamic nuclei of the rat. *J Comp Neurol* 2002; 448: 53-101.

[61] Antón-Bolaños N, Espinosa A, López-Bendito G. Developmental interactions between thalamus and cortex: a true love reciprocal story. *Curr Opin Neurobiol* 2018; 52: 33-41.

[62] Jones EG. A new view of specific and nonspecific thalamocortical connections. *Adv Neurol* 1998; 77: 49-71; discussion 72-3.

[63] Pouchelon G, Gambino F, Bellone C, et al. Modality-specific thalamocortical inputs instruct the identity of postsynaptic L4 neurons. *Nature* 2014; 511: 471-474.

[64] Zembrzycki A, Chou S-J, Ashery-Padan R, et al. Sensory cortex limits cortical maps and drives top-down plasticity in thalamocortical circuits. *Nat Neurosci* 2013; 16: 1060-1067.

[65] Mitrofanis J, Guillery RW. New views of the thalamic reticular nucleus in the adult and the developing brain. *Trends Neurosci* 1993; 16: 240-5.

[66] McCormick DA, Bal T. Sensory gating mechanisms of the thalamus. *Curr Opin Neurobiol* 1994; 4: 550-6.

[67] Nakajima M, Halassa MM. Thalamic control of functional cortical connectivity. *Curr Opin Neurobiol* 2017; 44: 127-131.

[68] Sherman SM, Guillery RW, Sherman SM. *Exploring the thalamus and its role in cortical function*. MIT Press, 2006.

[69] Sherman SM. Thalamic relay functions. *Prog Brain Res* 2001; 134: 51-69.

[70] Sherman SM. Functioning of Circuits Connecting Thalamus and Cortex. *Compr Physiol* 2017; 7: 713-739.

[71] Groenewegen HJ, Berendse HW. The specificity of the 'nonspecific' midline and intralaminar thalamic nuclei. *Trends Neurosci* 1994; 17: 52-7.

[72] Ramcharan EJ, Gnadt JW, Sherman SM. Higher-order thalamic relays burst more than first-order relays. *Proc Natl Acad Sci* 2005; 102: 12236-12241.

[73] Sherman SM. The thalamus is more than just a relay. *Curr Opin Neurobiol* 2007; 17: 417-422.

[74] Zhou J, Liu X, Song W, et al. Specific and nonspecific thalamocortical functional connectivity in normal and vegetative states. *Conscious Cogn* 2011; 20: 257-68.

[75] Jones EG. Thalamic circuitry and thalamocortical synchrony. *Philos Trans R Soc B Biol Sci* 2002; 357: 1659-1673.

[76] Lam Y-W, Sherman SM. Functional Organization of the Thalamic Input to the Thalamic Reticular Nucleus. *J Neurosci* 2011; 31: 6791-6799.

[77] Viviano JD, Schneider KA. Interhemispheric Interactions of the Human Thalamic Reticular Nucleus. *J Neurosci* 2015; 35: 2026-2032.

[78] Guillery RW, Harting JK. Structure and connections of the thalamic reticular nucleus: Advancing views over half a century. *J Comp Neurol* 2003; 463: 360-71.

[79] Yingling CD, Skinner JE. Selective regulation of thalamic sensory relay nuclei by nucleus reticularis thalami. *Electroencephalogr Clin Neurophysiol* 1976; 41: 476-82.

[80] Guillery RW, Feig SL, Lozsádi DA. Paying attention to the thalamic reticular nucleus. *Trends Neurosci* 1998; 21: 28-32.

[81] Jang SH, Lim HW, Yeo SS. The neural connectivity of the intralaminar

thalamic nuclei in the human brain: A diffusion tensor tractography study. *Neurosci Lett* 2014; 579: 140-144.

[82] Cicirata F, Angaut P, Serapide MF, et al. Functional organization of the direct and indirect projection via the reticularis thalami nuclear complex from the motor cortex to the thalamic nucleus ventralis lateralis. *Exp brain Res* 1990; 79: 325-37.

[83] Gonzalo-Ruiz A, Lieberman AR. Topographic organization of projections from the thalamic reticular nucleus to the anterior thalamic nuclei in the rat. *Brain Res Bull* 1995; 37: 17-35.

[84] Lozsádi DA. Organization of cortical afferents to the rostral, limbic sector of the rat thalamic reticular nucleus. *J Comp Neurol* 1994; 341: 520-33.

[85] Tai Y, Yi H, Ilinsky IA, et al. Nucleus reticularis thalami connections with the mediodorsal thalamic nucleus: a light and electron microscopic study in the monkey. *Brain Res Bull* 1995; 38: 475-88.

[86] McAlonan K, Brown VJ. The thalamic reticular nucleus: more than a sensory nucleus? *Neuroscientist* 2002; 8: 302-5.

[87] McAlonan K, Cavanaugh J, Wurtz RH. Attentional modulation of thalamic reticular neurons. *J Neurosci* 2006; 26: 4444-50.

[88] Min B-K. A thalamic reticular networking model of consciousness. *Theor Biol Med Model* 2010; 7: 10.

[89] Phillips JM, Kambi NA, Saalmann YB. A Subcortical Pathway for Rapid, Goal-Driven, Attentional Filtering. *Trends Neurosci* 2016; 39: 49-51.

[90] Wimmer RD, Schmitt LI, Davidson TJ, et al. Thalamic control of sensory selection in divided attention. *Nature* 2015; 526: 705-709.

[91] Saalmann YB. Intralaminar and medial thalamic influence on cortical synchrony, information transmission and cognition. *Front Syst Neurosci* 2014; 8: 83.

[92] de Medeiros Silva A, de Santana MAD, de Góis Morais PLA, et al. Serotonergic fibers distribution in the midline and intralaminar thalamic nuclei in the rock cavy (*Kerodon rupestris*). *Brain Res* 2014; 1586: 99-108.

[93] Kolaj M, Zhang L, Hermes MLHJ, et al. Intrinsic properties and neuropharmacology of midline paraventricular thalamic nucleus neurons. *Front Behav Neurosci* 2014; 8: 132.

[94] Pelzer EA, Melzer C, Timmermann L, et al. Basal ganglia and cerebellar interconnectivity within the human thalamus. *Brain Struct Funct* 2017; 222: 381-392.

[95] Varela C. Thalamic neuromodulation and its implications for executive networks. *Front Neural Circuits* 2014; 8: 69.

[96] Berendse HW, Groenewegen HJ. Restricted cortical termination fields of the midline and intralaminar thalamic nuclei in the rat. *Neuroscience* 1991; 42: 73-102.

[97] Benarroch EE. The midline and intralaminar thalamic nuclei: anatomic and functional specificity and implications in neurologic disease. *Neurology* 2008; 71: 944-9.

[98] Cornwall J, Phillipson OT. Afferent projections to the parafascicular thalamic nucleus of the rat, as shown by the retrograde transport of wheat germ agglutinin. *Brain Res Bull* 1988; 20: 139-50.

[99] Royce GJ, Bromley S, Gracco C. Subcortical projections to

the centromedian and parafascicular thalamic nuclei in the cat. *J Comp Neurol* 1991; 306: 129-55.

[100] Vertes RP, Linley SB, Hoover WB. Limbic circuitry of the midline thalamus. *Neurosci Biobehav Rev* 2015; 54: 89-107.

[101] Gummadavelli A, Motelow JE, Smith N, et al. Thalamic stimulation to improve level of consciousness after seizures: Evaluation of electrophysiology and behavior. *Epilepsia* 2015; 56: 114-124.

[102] Suffczynski P, Kalitzin S, Pfurtscheller G, et al. Computational model of thalamo-cortical networks: dynamical control of alpha rhythms in relation to focal attention. *Int J Psychophysiol* 2001; 43: 25-40.

[103] Crabtree JW, Isaac JTR. New intrathalamic pathways allowing modality-related and cross-modality switching in the dorsal thalamus. *J Neurosci* 2002; 22: 8754-61.

[104] Rodriguez-Sabate C, Llanos C, Morales I, et al. The functional connectivity of intralaminar thalamic nuclei in the human basal ganglia. *Hum Brain Mapp* 2015; 36: 1335-1347.

[105] Sadikot AF, Rymar V V. The primate centromedian-parafascicular complex: anatomical organization with a note on neuromodulation. *Brain Res Bull* 2009; 78: 122-30.

[106] Smith Y, Raju D V, Pare J-F, et al. The thalamostriatal system: a highly specific network of the basal ganglia circuitry. *Trends Neurosci* 2004; 27: 520-7.

[107] Vertes RP, Hoover WB, Rodriguez JJ. Projections of the central medial nucleus of the thalamus in the rat: node in cortical, striatal and limbic forebrain circuitry. *Neuroscience* 2012; 219: 120-36.

[108] Minamimoto T, Hori Y, Kimura M. Roles of the thalamic CM–PF complex—Basal ganglia circuit in externally driven rebias of action. *Brain Res Bull* 2009; 78: 75-79.

[109] Raeva SN. The role of the parafascicular complex (CM-Pf) of the human thalamus in the neuronal mechanisms of selective attention. *Neurosci Behav Physiol* 2006; 36: 287-95.

[110] Kinomura S, Larsson J, Gulyás B, et al. Activation by attention of the human reticular formation and thalamic intralaminar nuclei. *Science* 1996; 271: 512-5.

[111] Schlag-Rey M, Schlag J. Visuomotor functions of central thalamus in monkey. I. Unit activity related to spontaneous eye movements. *J Neurophysiol* 1984; 51: 1149-1174.

[112] Grunwerg BS, Krauthamer GM. Sensory responses of intralaminar thalamic neurons activated by the superior colliculus. *Exp brain Res* 1992; 88: 541-50.

[113] Biane JS, Takashima Y, Scanziani M, et al. Thalamocortical Projections onto Behaviorally Relevant Neurons Exhibit Plasticity during Adult Motor Learning. *Neuron* 2016; 89: 1173-1179.

[114] Schiff ND. Central thalamic deep brain stimulation for support of forebrain arousal regulation in the minimally conscious state. In: *Handbook of clinical neurology*, pp. 295-306.

[115] Schiff ND, Fins JJ. Deep brain stimulation and cognition: moving from animal to patient. *Curr Opin Neurol* 2007; 20: 638-642.

[116] Duan AR, Varela C, Zhang Y, et al. Delta Frequency Optogenetic Stimulation of the Thalamic Nucleus Reuniens Is Sufficient to Produce Working Memory Deficits: Relevance to

Schizophrenia. *Biol Psychiatry* 2015; 77: 1098-1107.

[117] Layfield DM, Patel M, Hallock H, et al. Inactivation of the nucleus reuniens/rhomboid causes a delay-dependent impairment of spatial working memory. *Neurobiol Learn Mem* 2015; 125: 163-167.

[118] Vertes RP. Major diencephalic inputs to the hippocampus. In: *Progress in brain research*, pp. 121-144.

[119] Vertes RP. Interactions among the medial prefrontal cortex, hippocampus and midline thalamus in emotional and cognitive processing in the rat. *Neuroscience* 2006; 142: 1-20.

[120] Cassel J-C, Pereira de Vasconcelos A, Loureiro M, et al. The reuniens and rhomboid nuclei: Neuroanatomy, electrophysiological characteristics and behavioral implications. *Prog Neurobiol* 2013; 111: 34-52.

[121] Çavdar S, Onat FY, Çakmak YÖ, et al. The pathways connecting the hippocampal formation, the thalamic reuniens nucleus and the thalamic reticular nucleus in the rat. *J Anat* 2008; 212: 249-256.

[122] Zikopoulos B, Barbas H. Circuits formultisensory integration and attentional modulation through the prefrontal cortex and the thalamic reticular nucleus in primates. *Rev Neurosci* 2007; 18: 417-38.

[123] Hsu DT, Price JL. Midline and intralaminar thalamic connections with the orbital and medial prefrontal networks in macaque monkeys. *J Comp Neurol* 2007; 504: 89-111.

[124] Jurik A, Auffenberg E, Klein S, et al. Roles of prefrontal cortex and paraventricular thalamus in affective and mechanical components of visceral nociception. *Pain* 2015; 156: 2479-2491.

[125] Kirouac GJ. Placing the paraventricular nucleus of the thalamus within the brain circuits that control behavior. *Neurosci Biobehav Rev* 2015; 56: 315-329.

[126] Penzo MA, Robert V, Tucciarone J, et al. The paraventricular thalamus controls a central amygdala fear circuit. *Nature* 2015; 519: 455-459.

[127] Dong X, Li S, Kirouac GJ. Collateralization of projections from the paraventricular nucleus of the thalamus to the nucleus accumbens, bed nucleus of the stria terminalis, and central nucleus of the amygdala. *Brain Struct Funct* 2017; 222: 3927-3943.

[128] Huang H, Ghosh P, van den Pol AN. Prefrontal cortex-projecting glutamatergic thalamic paraventricular nucleus-excited by hypocretin: a feedforward circuit that may enhance cognitive arousal. *J Neurophysiol* 2006; 95: 1656-68.

[129] Li S, Kirouac GJ. Sources of inputs to the anterior and posterior aspects of the paraventricular nucleus of the thalamus. *Brain Struct Funct* 2012; 217: 257-73.

[130] Vertes RP, Hoover WB. Projections of the paraventricular and paratenial nuclei of the dorsal midline thalamus in the rat. *J Comp Neurol* 2008; 508: 212-37.

[131] Rolls ET. Limbic systems for emotion and for memory, but no single limbic system. *Cortex* 2015; 62: 119-57.

[132] Luria A. Human brain and psychological processes.

[133] Boly M, Massimini M, Tsuchiya N, et al. Are the Neural Correlates of Consciousness in the Front or in the Back of the Cerebral Cortex? Clinical and Neuroimaging Evidence. *J Neurosci* 2017; 37: 9603-9613.

[134] Kirchgessner MA, Franklin AD, Callaway EM. Context-dependent and dynamic functional influence of corticothalamic pathways to first- and higher-order visual thalamus. *Proc Natl Acad Sci U S A* 2020; 117: 13066-13077.

[135] Storm JF, Boly M, Casali AG, et al. Consciousness Regained: Disentangling Mechanisms, Brain Systems, and Behavioral Responses. *J Neurosci* 2017; 37: 10882-10893.

[136] Mesulam MM. From sensation to cognition. *Brain* 1998; 121 (Pt 6): 1013-52.

[137] Dehaene S. The signatures of a conscious though. In: *Consciousness and the Brain*. New York: Penguin Books, 2014, pp. 115-160.

[138] Gaillard R, Dehaene S, Adam C, et al. Converging intracranial markers of conscious access. *PLoS Biol* 2009; 7: e61.

[139] Miller EK. The prefontral cortex and cognitive control. *Nat Rev Neurosci* 2000; 1: 59-65.

[140] Cole MW, Reynolds JR, Power JD, et al. Multi-task connectivity reveals flexible hubs for adaptive task control. *Nat Neurosci* 2013; 16: 1348-55.

[141] Boly M, Tshibanda L, Vanhaudenhuyse A, et al. Functional connectivity in the default network during resting state is preserved in a vegetative but not in a brain dead patient. *Hum Brain Mapp* 2009; 30: 2393-400.

[142] Buschman TJ, Miller EK. Top-Down Versus Bottom-Up Control of Attention in the Prefrontal and Posterior Parietal Cortices. *Science (80-)* 2007; 315: 1860-1862.

[143] Greicius MD, Supekar K, Menon V, et al. Resting-State Functional Connectivity Reflects Structural Connectivity in the Default Mode Network. *Cereb Cortex* 2009; 19: 72-78.

[144] Herbet G, Lafargue G, de Champfleur NM, et al. Disrupting posterior cingulate connectivity disconnects consciousness from the external environment. *Neuropsychologia* 2014; 56: 239-44.

[145] Raichle ME. The Brain's Default Mode Network. *Annu Rev Neurosci* 2015; 38: 433-447.

[146] Raichle ME, MacLeod AM, Snyder AZ, et al. A default mode of brain function. *Proc Natl Acad Sci* 2001; 98: 676-682.

[147] Fox MD, Raichle ME. Spontaneous fluctuations in brain activity observed with functional magnetic resonance imaging. *Nat Rev Neurosci* 2007; 8: 700-711.

[148] Fransson P, Marrelec G. The precuneus/posterior cingulate cortex plays a pivotal role in the default mode network: Evidence from a partial correlation network analysis. *Neuroimage* 2008; 42: 1178-84.

[149] Greicius MD, Menon V. Default-mode activity during a passive sensory task: uncoupled from deactivation but impacting activation. *J Cogn Neurosci* 2004; 16: 1484-92.

[150] Shulman GL, Fiez JA, Corbetta M, et al. Common Blood Flow Changes across Visual Tasks: II. Decreases in Cerebral Cortex. *J Cogn Neurosci* 1997; 9: 648-663.

[151] Greicius MD, Krasnow B, Reiss AL, et al. Functional connectivity in the resting brain: A network analysis of the default mode hypothesis. *Proc Natl Acad Sci* 2003; 100: 253-258.

[152] Mason MF, Norton MI, Van Horn JD, et al. Wandering Minds:

The Default Network and Stimulus-Independent Thought. *Science (80-)* 2007; 315: 393-395.

[153] Andrews-Hanna JR, Smallwood J, Spreng RN. The default network and self-generated thought: component processes, dynamic control, and clinical relevance. *Ann N Y Acad Sci* 2014; 1316: 29-52.

[154] Axelrod V, Rees G, Bar M. The default network and the combination of cognitive processes that mediate self-generated thought. *Nat Hum Behav* 2017; 1: 896-910.

[155] Kucyi A, Esterman M, Riley CS, et al. Spontaneous default network activity reflects behavioral variability independent of mind-wandering. *Proc Natl Acad Sci* 2016; 113: 13899-13904.

[156] Bellana B, Liu Z-X, Diamond NB, et al. Similarities and differences in the default mode network across rest, retrieval, and future imagining. *Hum Brain Mapp* 2017; 38: 1155-1171.

[157] Monge ZA, Wing EA, Stokes J, et al. Search and recovery of autobiographical and laboratory memories: Shared and distinct neural components. *Neuropsychologia* 2018; 110: 44-54.

[158] Henry JD, Crawford JR, Phillips LH. Verbal fluency performance in dementia of the Alzheimer's type: a meta-analysis. *Neuropsychologia* 2004; 42: 1212-1222.

[159] Philippi CL, Tranel D, Duff M, et al. Damage to the default mode network disrupts autobiographical memory retrieval. *Soc Cogn Affect Neurosci* 2015; 10: 318-326.

[160] Smith V, Mitchell DJ, Duncan J. Role of the Default Mode Network in Cognitive Transitions. *Cereb Cortex* 2018; 28: 3685-3696.

[161] Snyder AZ, Raichle ME. A brief history of the resting state: the Washington University perspective. *Neuroimage* 2012; 62: 902-10.

[162] Han K, Chapman SB, Krawczyk DC. Disrupted Intrinsic Connectivity among Default, Dorsal Attention, and Frontoparietal Control Networks in Individuals with Chronic Traumatic Brain Injury. *J Int Neuropsychol Soc* 2016; 22: 263-279.

[163] Long J, Xie Q, Ma Q, et al. Distinct Interactions between Fronto-Parietal and Default Mode Networks in Impaired Consciousness. *Sci Rep* 2016; 6: 38866.

[164] Finc K, Bonna K, Lewandowska M, et al. Transition of the functional brain network related to increasing cognitive demands. *Hum Brain Mapp* 2017; 38: 3659-3674.

[165] Niendam TA, Laird AR, Ray KL, et al. Meta-analytic evidence for a superordinate cognitive control network subserving diverse executive functions. *Cogn Affect Behav Neurosci* 2012; 12: 241-68.

[166] Spreng RN, Stevens WD, Chamberlain JP, et al. Default network activity, coupled with the frontoparietal control network, supports goal-directed cognition. *Neuroimage* 2010; 53: 303-17.

[167] Vincent JL, Kahn I, Snyder AZ, et al. Evidence for a Frontoparietal Control System Revealed by Intrinsic Functional Connectivity. *J Neurophysiol* 2008; 100: 3328-3342.

[168] Vossel S, Geng JJ, Fink GR. Dorsal and ventral attention systems: distinct neural circuits but collaborative roles. *Neuroscientist* 2014; 20: 150-9.

[169] Menon V. Salience Network. In: *Brain mapping : an encyclopedic reference*. Amsterdam: Elsevier Inc, 2015, pp. 597-611.

[170] Chen AC, Oathes DJ, Chang C, et al. Causal interactions between fronto-parietal central executive and default-mode networks in humans. *Proc Natl Acad Sci* 2013; 110: 19944-19949.

[171] Corbetta M, Shulman GL. CONTROL OF GOAL-DIRECTED AND STIMULUS-DRIVEN ATTENTION IN THE BRAIN. *Nat Rev Neurosci* 2002; 3: 215-229.

[172] Fox MD, Snyder AZ, Vincent JL, et al. From The Cover: The human brain is intrinsically organized into dynamic, anticorrelated functional networks. *Proc Natl Acad Sci* 2005; 102: 9673-9678.

[173] Sridharan D, Levitin DJ, Menon V. A critical role for the right fronto-insular cortex in switching between central-executive and default-mode networks. *Proc Natl Acad Sci* 2008; 105: 12569-12574.

[174] Zhou Y, Friston KJ, Zeidman P, et al. The Hierarchical Organization of the Default, Dorsal Attention and Salience Networks in Adolescents and Young Adults. *Cereb Cortex* 2018; 28: 726-737.

[175] (Bud) Craig AD. How do you feel — now? The anterior insula and human awareness. *Nat Rev Neurosci* 2009; 10: 59-70.

[176] Fox MD, Corbetta M, Snyder AZ, et al. Spontaneous neuronal activity distinguishes human dorsal and ventral attention systems. *Proc Natl Acad Sci U S A* 2006; 103: 10046-51.

[177] Gogolla N, Takesian AE, Feng G, et al. Sensory integration in mouse insular cortex reflects GABA circuit maturation. *Neuron* 2014; 83: 894-905.

[178] Menon V, Uddin LQ. Saliency, switching, attention and control: a network model of insula function. *Brain Struct Funct* 2010; 214: 655-67.

[179] Sonuga-Barke EJS, Castellanos FX. Spontaneous attentional fluctuations in impaired states and pathological conditions: a neurobiological hypothesis. *Neurosci Biobehav Rev* 2007; 31: 977-86.

[180] Anticevic A, Cole MW, Murray JD, et al. The role of default network deactivation in cognition and disease. *Trends Cogn Sci* 2012; 16: 584-592.

[181] Dosenbach NUF, Fair DA, Miezin FM, et al. Distinct brain networks for adaptive and stable task control in humans. *Proc Natl Acad Sci* 2007; 104: 11073-11078.

[182] Crone JS, Ladurner G, Höller Y, et al. Deactivation of the default mode network as a marker of impaired consciousness: an fMRI study. *PLoS One* 2011; 6: e26373.

[183] Supekar K, Cai W, Krishnadas R, et al. Dysregulated Brain Dynamics in a Triple-Network Saliency Model of Schizophrenia and Its Relation to Psychosis. *Biol Psychiatry*. Epub ahead of print 1 August 2018. DOI: 10.1016/j.biopsych.2018.07.020.

[184] Fan D, Liao F, Wang Q. The pacemaker role of thalamic reticular nucleus in controlling spike-wave discharges and spindles. *Chaos An Interdiscip J Nonlinear Sci* 2017; 27: 073103.

[185] Spreng RN, Schacter DL. Default network modulation and large-scale network interactivity in healthy young and old adults. *Cereb Cortex* 2012; 22: 2610-21.

[186] Spreng RN, Sepulcre J, Turner GR, et al. Intrinsic architecture underlying the relations among the default, dorsal attention, and frontoparietal control networks of the human brain. *J Cogn Neurosci* 2013; 25: 74-86.

[187] Seeley WW, Menon V, Schatzberg AF, et al. Dissociable intrinsic connectivity networks for salience processing and executive control. *J Neurosci* 2007; 27: 2349-56.

[188] León-Carrión J, León-Dominguez U, Halper J, et al. Restoring cortical connectivity directionality and synchronization is essential to treating disorder of consciousness. *Curr Pharm Des* 2014; 20: 4268-74.

[189] Amico E, Marinazzo D, Di Perri C, et al. Mapping the functional connectome traits of levels of consciousness. *Neuroimage* 2017; 148: 201-211.

[190] Dietrich A. Functional neuroanatomy of altered states of consciousness: the transient hypofrontality hypothesis. *Conscious Cogn* 2003; 12: 231-56.

[191] Parras GG, Nieto-Diego J, Carbajal G V., et al. Neurons along the auditory pathway exhibit a hierarchical organization of prediction error. *Nat Commun* 2017; 8: 2148.

[192] Dehaene S, Changeux J-P, Naccache L, et al. Conscious, preconscious, and subliminal processing: a testable taxonomy. *Trends Cogn Sci* 2006; 10: 204-11.

Chapter 6

Interplay between Primary Cortical Areas and Crossmodal Plasticity

Christian Xerri and Yoh'i Zennou-Azogui

Abstract

Perceptual representations are built through multisensory interactions underpinned by dense anatomical and functional neural networks that interconnect primary and associative cortical areas. There is compelling evidence that primary sensory cortical areas do not work in segregation, but play a role in early processes of multisensory integration. In this chapter, we firstly review previous and recent literature showing how multimodal interactions between primary cortices may contribute to refining perceptual representations. Secondly, we discuss findings providing evidence that, following peripheral damage to a sensory system, multimodal integration may promote sensory substitution in deprived cortical areas and favor compensatory plasticity in the spared sensory cortices.

Keywords: multisensory convergence, crossmodal processing, sensory loss, intersensory substitution

1. Introduction

The brain's ability to generate a rich and unambiguous representation of the world requires the multimodal integration of sensory signals often co-occurring in time and space. A crucial issue is how the brain integrates the separate elements of an object perceived through individual sensory channels (vision, audition, touch, etc.) in order not only to improve detection and discrimination and evaluate crossmodal congruency, but also to form a unified percept. Over the last decades, a growing number of studies have challenged the traditional view of the sensory neocortex as a parcellation of highly specialized primary areas, each being exclusively dedicated to the integration and processing of a unique sensory modality. An ancillary conception is that signals conveyed through unisensory streams mainly converge and interact in higher-order association regions of the temporal and parietal cortex in which multisensory integration culminates. Accordingly, these cortical regions tuned to integrate increasingly complex sensory signals send divergent projections back to early sensory areas to exert modulatory feedback on their constituent neurons. However, this hierarchical model of multisensory integration has been reappraised in view of accumulating evidence over recent decades that primary sensory cortical areas are anatomically and functionally interconnected. There is increasing awareness that multisensory integration starts in lower sensory areas, presumably via thalamo-cortical and direct cortico-cortical connections [1–3] (macaque; ferret) ([4, 5], for reviews). Hence, it is of primary interest to unravel how heteromodal inputs interplaying with the dominant modality in primary sensory areas may contribute to improving perception. In addition, a major issue is to determine how crossmodal plasticity subserves functional compensation and behavioral recovery after the loss or impairment of a sensory organ, or following cortical damage. This review chapter has a double focus, firstly on the interplay between primary sensory cortices in normal condition, and secondly on crossmodal plasticity operating in primary and higher-order cortical areas following sensory loss.

2. Subcortical and intracortical connectivity between primary sensory areas

There is anatomical evidence that crossmodal inputs to primary cortical areas can be conveyed through thalamo-cortical or cortico-cortical projection fibers. There is, however, only scarce anatomical evidence for heteromodal convergence from auditory, visual and somatosensory thalamic nuclei to A1, V1 and S1 [6] (gerbil). By contrast, cortico-cortical connections underpinning plurimodal interplay between these cortical areas are well documented. Tract-tracing methods have revealed the existence of visual-somatosensory projections from V2 to areas 1/3b in S1, and somatosensory projections from S2 to A1 [2] (marmoset). Direct cortico-cortical connections between A1, V1 and S1 have been identified [1, 7] (macaque; cat). It has been shown that V1 projects mainly to S1, but receives a moderate amount of projections from A1 and S1, while A1 sends more projections to V1 than S1, but receives sparse projections from these two areas [8, 9] (mouse). These findings indicate that the connectivity network between A1, S1 and V1 is asymmetric. Overall, both thalamocortical and corticocortical connections may contribute to the occurrence of short-latency responses to heteromodal inputs reported in these area [10–17] (monkey; human).

In the model of hierarchical organization of cortical connectivity, it is generally assumed that feedforward connections convey sensory information to higher order areas, whereas feedback connections modulate neural activity in lower-level cortical areas [18, 19] (macaque; cat). This model is somewhat challenged by retrograde tracing studies investigating the microcircuitry of reciprocal connections between primary cortical areas. These studies have shown that A1 and S1 project in a feedback manner to V1, while V1 to A1 projections are of feedforward type and V1 to S1 are mostly lateral [8, 9] (mouse). In addition, A1 and S1 are linked by reciprocal feedback projections [6] (gerbil). Hence, the available evidence suggests that connection patterns between primary sensory cortices are not at the same levels in the neural network. Furthermore, based on the labeling of reciprocal connections between V1 and S1 and the characterization of the size and laminar density of axonal swellings, it was concluded that S1 receives a stronger driver input fromV1 and that S1 inputs to V1 have a predominant modulatory influence [9] (mouse). Regarding the projections from the auditory cortex to V1, both types of input have been identified with, however, a clear dominance of small caliber axons bearing modulator boutons [8] (mouse).

Somatosensory-auditory interactions have been found at low-level of multisensory integration. Cutaneous responses were recorded in the caudo-medial auditory cortex, with a feedforward laminar activation profile. The initial excitatory response was located in layer 4, then followed by responses in the extragranular laminae (layers 2, 3, 5 and 6), in contrast with feedback and lateral activation profiles beginning in the extragranular laminae [20] (macaque).

The intricate connectivity between unimodal primary cortical areas favors crossmodal interplay in the early stage of multisensory integration, presumably through feedforward and feedback connections [21] (for a review). The question arises whether heteromodal connections between low-level sensory cortices exert a global modulatory influence on ongoing firing or more selectively contribute to shaping the neuronal response characteristics in primary sensory areas.

3. Neurophysiological mechanisms of multimodal integration in primary sensory areas

Concurrent stimuli of sensory organs coactivate primary cortical areas and generate reciprocal influences contributing to the process of multimodal integration. It is noticeable that the bulk of studies on multisensory integration in early cortical areas have focused on the interplay between the visual and auditory cortices.

3.1 Visual-auditory interactions

Activation of A1 neurons by noise bursts was found to induce GABAergic inhibition of supragranular pyramidal cells in V1, via cortico-cortical connections, leading to a reduced synaptic and spike activity upon bimodal stimulation [10] (mouse). Furthermore, this acoustic stimulation decreased behavioral responses to a dim flash, likely through GABAergic inhibition in V1, as this effect was prevented by acute blockade of $GABA_A$ and $GABA_B$ receptors. The authors concluded that salient auditory stimuli degrade potentially distracting sensory processing in the visual cortex. This finding was corroborated by an *in vitro* electrophysiological study showing that layer 1 and layer 2/3 inhibitory neurons in V1 receive direct excitatory inputs from A1 [22] (mouse). Along the same lines, intrinsic signal imaging aimed at simultaneously recording visuotopic maps in V1 and tonotopic maps in A1, showed that a high activation of A1 suppresses visually evoked responses in V1 [5] (mouse). As a result, under bimodal stimulation the global effect of auditory inputs to V1 was such that the neuronal firing averaged across all visual orientations was weaker. Nevertheless, the orientation selectivity of V1 excitatory neurons in layer 2/layer 3 was found to be sharpened by concurrent sound signals or optogenetic activation of A1 to V1 projections [22] (mouse). Indeed, auditory signals increased the neuronal responses at the preferred visual orientation, and decreased responses at the orthogonal orientation, with a stronger impact at lower visual contrast. Tracing data showed that axons from A1 layer 5 to V1 neurons mainly terminated in superficial layers and activated layer 1 inhibitory neurons. The sharpening effect was very likely mediated by a combination of inhibitory and disinhibitory circuits, since layer 1 neurons in V1 being excited by sound, they presumably suppressed layer 2/layer 3 pyramidal cell responses, but also inhibited other inhibitory neurons in layer 2/layer 3, thereby globally contributing to increasing the firing rate of the pyramidal cells at their preferred orientation tuning. A two-photon calcium imaging study showed that when visual and auditory stimulus features are temporally congruent, neurons in V1 exhibit a balanced pattern of response enhancement and suppression compared with unimodal visual stimuli. Temporally incongruent tones or white-noise bursts in paired audiovisual stimuli mainly produce suppressive responses across the neuronal population, in particular when the visual stimulus contrast is high [23] (mouse). Neuronal mechanisms of visual–auditory integration appear to be dependent upon the behavioral context. A study investigating the modulation of V1 neurons by auditory stimuli showed no difference in the latency or strength of visual responses in monkeys trained to a passive central fixation, while a visual–auditory stimulus was presented in the periphery [24] (monkey). By contrast, a significant reduction in latency was observed when the animal was required to orient its gaze toward the visual–auditory stimulus. This finding suggests that projections from the auditory cortex to V1 contribute to reducing the response time of head orientation during a foveation movement toward a peripheral sound source.

There is also convincing evidence that vision impacts neuronal coding in the primary auditory cortex. Neurons sensitive to visual stimulation in A1 convey more information about stimuli in their spike trains than neurons sensitive to either auditory or visual stimuli presented alone [3] (ferret). An intriguing study revealed that adding congruent visual signals to auditory ones enhanced the weak auditory responses, had no effect on intermediate responses and suppressed strong responses [25] (macaque). In this study, measurement of the amount of information contained in visual and auditory responses showed that bimodal stimuli yielded more information provided by firing rates and spike timing than unimodal ones, but that the suppressed responses carried more information than the increased responses. This information gain was due to a reduced variability of the suppressed responses, whereas the variability of the enhanced responses was increased. The authors proposed that enhanced, but less reliable responses may be involved in detecting rare or faint sensory events, while suppressed, more reliable responses may be used to represent detailed characteristics of sensory environment. Interestingly, a recent study suggests that in layers 5 and 6 of the auditory cortex, a primary locus of visual–auditory convergence, visual signals convey the presence and timing of a salient stimulus rather than specifics about that stimulus, i.e. auditory responses are not orientation-tuned to visual gratings unlike visual cortex responses [26] (mouse).

3.2 Somatosensory-auditory interactions

Besides the notion that crossmodal interactions are reflected by changes in firing rates, the synchronization of neural signals has been proposed as a key mechanism for multisensory integration in distributed networks [27]. In this regard, it is relevant to mention a study exploring the influence of somatosensory inputs on the activity of A1 neurons using laminar current source density and multiunit recordings. The findings show that somatosensory inputs elicited by median nerve stimulation amplify the neuronal responses evoked by auditory inputs during a high-excitability phase of ongoing local neuronal oscillations and suppress those occurring during a low-excitability phase in the supragranular layers [28] (macaque). Further analysis indicated that this effect was mainly due to a somatosensory-induced phase resetting of auditory oscillations to an optimal excitability phase enhancing the ensemble response of temporally coherent auditory inputs.

Neurons in the posterior region of A1 display cutaneous receptive fields specifically located on the head and neck, which are in spatial register with the auditory receptive fields [29] (macaque). This result supports the view that the posterior auditory cortex may be the site for spatial-movement processing, analogous to the "where pathway" in the parietal stream of the visual system [30, 31] (macaque). A fMRI study documented a supra-additive integration of touch and auditory stimulation in a cortical region posterior and lateral to A1 [32] (macaque). This integration process was more prominent for temporally coincident bimodal stimuli and for less effective stimuli, in conformity with the principle of "inverse effectiveness".

3.3 Visual-somatosensory interactions

It is worth reporting a fMRI study aiming to compare cortical activation in response to matching versus non-matching visual–haptic texture information in a task that did not require cognitive evaluation of roughness [33] (human). The results show an increased BOLD response in V1 when a dot pattern was presented in both visual and haptic conditions, all the more so whenever visual information matched haptic texture information. In addition, parametric BOLD signal variations with varying texture characteristics were recorded in both primary visual and somatosensory cortices. This study confirms that haptic information can modulate visual information processing at an early stage. A hierarchical feedback of top-down influences from higher sensory areas on early sensory cortices could account for the observed BOLD effects. However, according to the authors this is unlikely, as only matching visual–haptic texture information induced a parametric modulation of the BOLD response in the contralateral somatosensory cortex. An alternative, more plausible, interpretation of the crossmodal texture effects would be direct or indirect cortico-cortical connections between primary areas. This explanation is compatible with haptic texture information flowing from S1 to V1 [34] (human).

Interestingly, a shrinkage of cutaneous receptive fields in areas 3b and 1 has been recorded when tactile and visual stimulations were concomitant, both during physical touch perception and touch observation [35] (human). This sharpening of coactivated receptive fields that reflects a suppressive interaction between tactile and visual cues, presumably occurring through a GABAergic modulation of intracortical inhibition in S1, is expected to improve tactile acuity (for reviews, see [36, 37]). The functional relevance of this finding was highlighted by a study reporting that viewing the hand increased the suppression of the P50 evoked potential due to simultaneous electrical stimulation of adjacent fingers and enhanced tactile acuity in a task of grating orientation discrimination [38] (human). Furthermore, a recent ultra-high-resolution fMRI study provided evidence for a spatially specific visual convergence onto S1. Neurons within the somatotopically organized cutaneous representation of the fingers in areas 3b and 1 were activated by the subject observing his fingers being touched, or the fingers of another person receiving similar tactile stimulation [39]. The visually-driven map was topographically and temporally precise and was found to be in register with the cutaneous map. Further investigations of the neuron characteristics within area 3b and area 1 are required to determine whether or not this area may contribute to distinguishing perceived touch from observed touch.

3.4 Vestibular-somatosensory interactions

The vestibular cortex differs from other sensory cortices in that vestibular signals are distributed in an extensive network of cortical regions [40–42]. A whole-brain electrophysiological investigation using galvanic vestibular stimulation and fMRI mapping described the cortical projections of vestibular inputs to functionally diverse cortical regions that included S1 [43] (rat). In addition, a more recent investigation revealed that the optogenetic stimulation of the medial vestibular nucleus neurons elicited bilateral fMRI activations in the sensorimotor cortices and their thalamic nuclei [44] (rat). Nevertheless, which region of S1 receives vestibular inputs and how the bimodal interplay occurs has not yet been investigated. In a recent study in rat, we reasoned that the vestibulo-somatosensory convergence in S1 could occur in the cortical zones of the paw representations that would be congruent with the functional role of these inputs in posturo-locomotor regulation. Accordingly, we evaluated the immediate effects of a complete unilateral vestibular neurectomy on the response properties of S1 neurons in the hindpaw cutaneous representations [45]. We found that the acute deafferentation immediately induces a bilateral expansion of the cutaneous receptive fields that exclusively concerned those located on the plantar skin surfaces. A corrolary effect consisted of a dedifferentiation of the topographic organization of the cortical maps representing these surfaces (**Figure 1**). However, this somatotopy disruption was relatively less pronounced for the representation of ipsilesional hindpaw, consistently with the contralateral predominance of vestibulo-thalamic projections [46, 47] (cat). The rapid deafferentation-induced expansion of cutaneous receptive field indicates that in intact animals, vestibular inputs exert a suppressive effect onto synaptic inputs driving cutaneous responses in S1.

It is well documented that cortical maps are dynamically reshaped through ongoing adjustments in the balance of excitatory and inhibitory influences on their constituent neurons. Hence, it is very likely that the receptive field enlargement induced by the vestibular loss results from a disinhibition process, possibly via thalamo-cortical inputs on S1 inhibitory interneurons or direct cortico-cortical connections. It has long been argued that intracortical inhibition plays a key role in controlling the spatial selectivity of cortical neurons through segregation of broad sets of converging synaptic inputs. Consistently, studies have reported a substantial enlargement of the cutaneous receptive field of somatosensory cortical neurons when GABA-mediated local inhibition was antagonized by an intracortical bicuculine injection [48–50] (cat; racoon), whereas injection of baclofen, a selective agonist for the $GABA_A$ receptors, induced a shrinkage of these receptive fields [51] (rat). A release of afferent-driven intracortical tonic inhibition results in an enhanced effectiveness of convergent cutaneous inputs. Therefore, this could be a most likely mechanism for rapid unmasking of previously subthreshold afferent connections reflected by the rapid expansion of cutaneous receptive field of S1 neurons following the loss of vestibular inputs. Our results extend previous findings, already mentioned in the present review, showing that auditory inputs to V1 decrease visually induced activity (mouse), while acute hearing loss releases the inhibitory effects of A1 neurons on visually elicited responses in V1 and leads to a concomitant increase in V1 activation [52] (mouse). As also previously noted, auditory stimulation sharpens the orientation selectivity of V1 neurons [22] (mouse). Collectively, the available evidence supports the view that, in normal conditions, cross modal modulation between primary cortical cortices may act to improve the tuning of neuronal response properties in these areas. In our study, the postlesion expansion of cutaneous RF was selectively located on the hindpaw plantar skin surfaces. Hence, we hypothesize that, in normal conditions, the vestibular influences on the S1 cortex could improve tactile acuity during perceptually guided posturo-locomotor adjustments.

3.5 Crossmodal interplay in transitory cortical regions bridging primary sensory areas

The main focus of the present review is on multimodal integration in primary cortical areas. Nonetheless, while considering low-level crossmodal interplay, it is relevant to mention findings related to multimodal convergence and integration in transitional zones lying between primary areas. Visual and somatosensory inputs converge and interact in a graded multisensory zone forming a narrow strip within the associative parietal cortex (APC) of rodent. Previous findings analyzing current source density [53] (rat), or using calcium imaging [54] (mouse) or

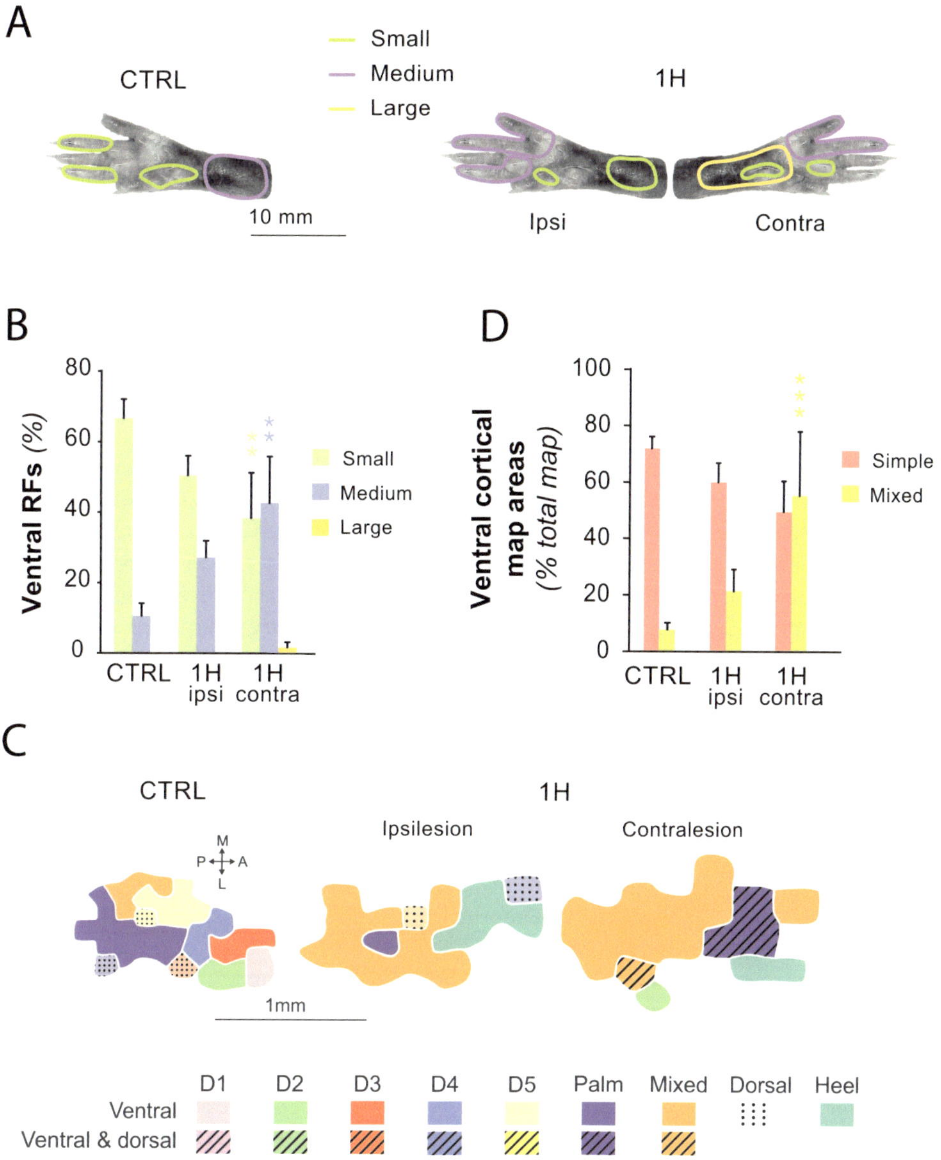

Figure 1.
*Immediate effects of unilateral vestibular neurectomy on hindpaw cutaneous representation in S1. (A) Typical receptive fields (RFs) recorded in the S1 cortex and located on hindpaw glabrous skin surfaces of an intact rat (CTRL, left panel) and after double mapping, on ipsilesional (ipsi) and contralesional (contra) hindpaws one hour after unilateral vestibular neurectomy (UVN) (1H, right panel). In green: small size RFs covering less than 10% of the total skin surface of the paw; in purple: medium size RFs >10% and <40% of the paw surface; in yellow: large size RFs including more than 40% of the paw surface. (B) Distribution of plantar cutaneous RF recorded in CTRL and UVN rats. The height of each area of the stacked histogram represents the mean proportion of RFs falling into each category (green: small; purple: medium; yellow: large RFs). (C) Representative electrophysiological cortical maps obtained from an intact rat (CTRL: left panel) and from two rats in which ipsilesional and contralesional hindpaw maps were obtained starting 1 hour after UVN (1H, right panel). The map remodeling was accounted for by the expansion of plantar cutaneous RF illustrated in A-B. Note the drastic dedifferentiation of the somatotopic maps. Simple areas correspond to neurons with RF located on the ventral or dorsal aspect of individual fingers, or encompassing palmar pads. Mixed areas correspond to neurons displaying enlarged RFs extending beyond the somatotopic regions observed in prelesion hindlimb maps, i.e. RFs on 2 or more skin territories of the hindpaw. (D) Stacked histogram showing the relative mean areas of the different map regions, normalized with respect to the total hindlimb area. These relative areas are color-coded (green: simple area; purple: mixed area). **: $P < 0.01$; ***: $P < 0.001$ (comparisons with control values); (Kruskal Wallis analysis and Dunnett's post-hoc test). Vertical bars illustrate standard errors of the means (SEM). Hairy skin RFs and representational zones were not altered after acute UVN [modified from Facchini et al. (in press)].*

voltage-sensitive dye imaging (VSDI) described this region as heteromodal [55] (rat). In addition, a gradual merging of modalities from the borders of the primary cortices to the middle of the APC strip has been reported [54] (mouse). Using optical imaging combined with laminar electrophysiological recordings, it was observed that both inputs elicited similar response patterns in this cortical zone [53] (rat) However, current source density analysis of event-related potentials revealed a supra-additive interaction of subthreshold activity when the somatosensory response preceded the visual response, whereas a sub-linear summation was induced by reversing the stimulus order. This finding suggests an asymmetry in the excitation-inhibition balance mediated by the underlying connectivity network, that may be consistent with the observation that visual responses were located deeper than somatosensory responses. The laminar pattern of these visual-somatosensory interactions and the fact that they vanished upon GABAergic silencing of local post-synaptic activity suggest their intracortical origin.

In a recent study, we investigated the neural processing of visual and somatosensory motion cues in individual neurons of the APC [56] (rat). The animals were exposed to moving visual gratings presented in different directions, with various motion speeds, and to air puffs deflecting bilaterally all the whiskers in the antero-posterior (backward) or postero-anterior (forward) directions. When delivered simultaneously, visual and tactile stimuli could be either in the same or opposite direction (congruent or incongruent). We used both voltage-sensitive dye imaging to identify the cortical zone of convergence of tactile and visual afferents, and single-unit recordings to investigate the uni- and bimodal processing of these inputs. We showed the convergence of visual and tactile information, both in layer 2/3 as revealed by VSDI, and in layer 4, as demonstrated by the single-unit recordings. Both whisker deflections and visual moving gratings evoked neural responses in the APC, with similar magnitudes, reflecting the convergence of equally weighted visual and somatosensory information (**Figure 2**). The majority of recorded cells were bimodal with about 50% exhibiting a directional congruence for the stimulus orientations tested, which strongly points to a potential role of the APC in heteromodal sensory integration. A machine learning approach revealed that the integration of the visual-tactile motion stimuli relies predominantly on the bimodal population, as performing decoding on the unimodal neurons did not yield accuracies above chance. In addition, we found that visual neurons in APC selectively respond to the direction (about 50%) and speed (about 30%) of visual grating motion, while somatosensory neurons display a direction selectivity for whisker stimulation (about 60%). Like in the study mentioned above [53], a temporal dissociation was observed between somatosensory and visual responses, both in the supragranular and granular layers, as the somatosensory stimulations evoked earlier responses than did the visual stimulations. This finding underscores the importance of timing in multimodal integration, and is consistent with the view that whiskers information predominantly relates to fast changing contacts with objects or congeners, while vision mainly provides information about the physical and social environment that likely facilitates the interpretation of somatosensory information. It is plausible that APC is designed as a hub in which multisensory motion information is integrated to contribute to elaborating in higher-order areas a supramodal percept guiding purposeful behavior. Interestingly, these animal studies are consistent with human investigations showing the existence of a multisensory homunculus posterior to S1, along the postcentral sulcus, that overlaps the most anterior retinotopic map with a topographic alignment of tactile and visual representations [57, 58]. The authors proposed that these multisensory topographically organized maps may play a pivotal role in perception and cognition related to peripersonal space.

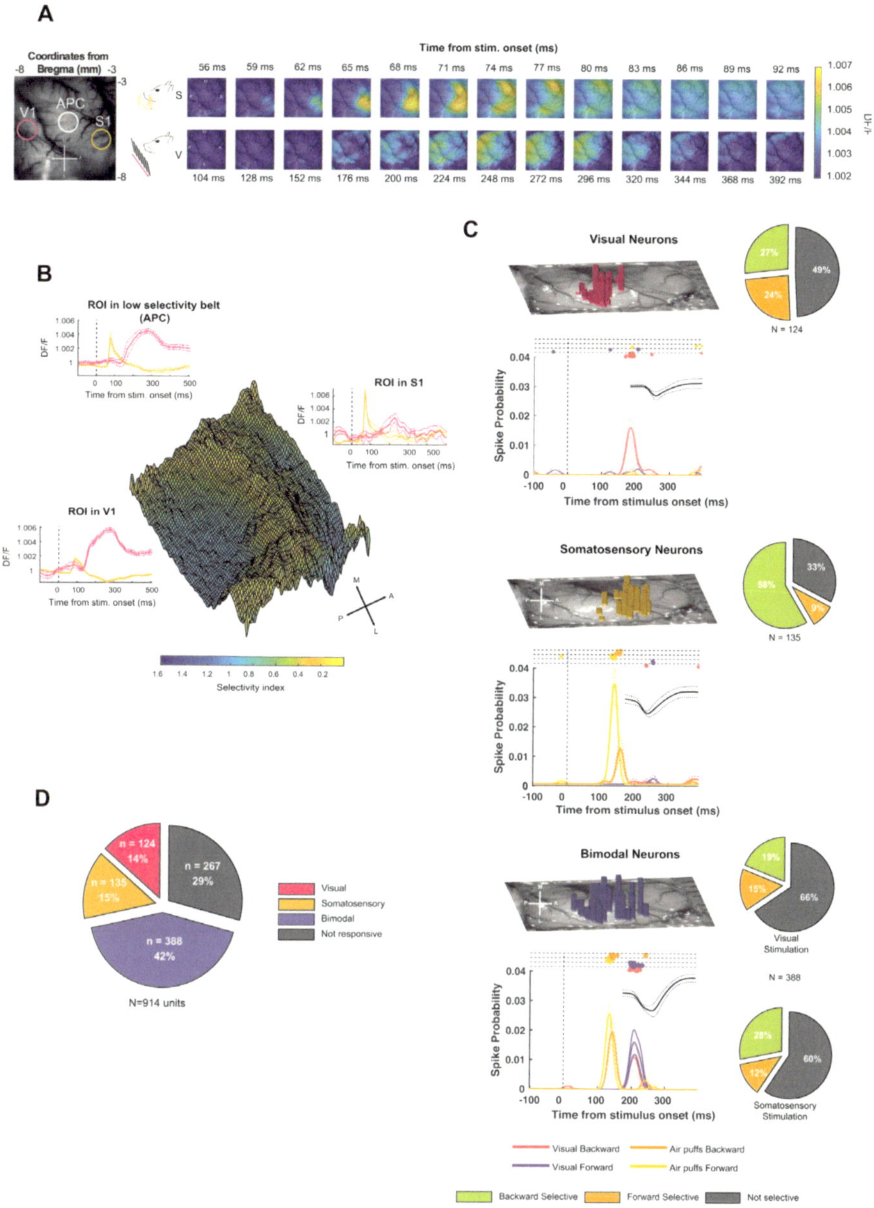

Figure 2.

Convergence of visual and somatosensory inputs in the associative parietal cortex (APC). (A) Example of cortical activation dynamics evoked by somatosensory (upper row) or visual (lower row) stimulation revealed by voltage-sensitive-dye imaging. The latency to the somatosensory stimulation (60 – 90 ms) is shorter than to the visual stimulation (150 – 350 ms). The value in ms indicate the time after stimulation onset. (B) Example of mean DF/F over time. Time course of responses to the unimodal stimuli, in V1, S1 and APC with a 3D representation of selectivity indices. For each pixel of the acquisition window the colormap depicts the level of selectivity. The low selectivity belt (yellow) is characterized by comparable levels of activation ("ROI in low selectivity belt (APC)" plot), while high selectivity indices (blue) are observed in S1 and V1. (C) Spatial distribution of the recorded neurons corresponding to the visual, somatosensory and bimodal conditions for a representative animal. The heights of the histograms represent the proportions of neurons recorded at the corresponding cortical sites. The proportion of direction selective cells in the neuronal populations is indicated (backward, green; forward, yellow; not selective, gray). Examples of a recorded unit significantly responding only to the backward visual stimulus (pink line), a unit responding to both air puff directions, with a larger spiking probability to the forward direction and a bimodal neuron that responds to all 4 conditions. The inset presents the unit's waveform. The spiking probabilities to each condition are represented as a function of time from stimulus onset. Note the latency shift existing in neuronal response to visual and somatosensory conditions in the neurons recorded in APC. (D) Proportions of visual (pink), somatosensory (yellow), bimodal (blue) and non-responsive (gray) neurons recorded in the APC (N = 914) (modified from Caron-Guyon et al. [56]).

The set of studies reviewed highlights the broad panoply of connectivity patterns and functional interactions between primary areas that underpin a flexible cooperation at an early stage of sensory processing. Tentatively, we propose that early crossmodal interactions in primary areas contribute to refining and sharpening neural response tuning adapted to improving "immediate" perception and eliminating perceptual ambiguity. This perceptual optimization could occur through rapid neurophysiological mechanisms operating in the corticocortical circuitry (e. g., local suppressive inhibition, sub-additive or supra-additive integration, oscillatory entrainment of neuronal networks) and serve automated behavioral responses. According to this view, cognitive influences exerted onto higher-order cortical integration areas, operating through relatively slower mechanisms, would adaptively modulate the early multimodal integration to fulfill a more complex integration processing influenced by attention and motivation so as to adjust perception to a continuously changing behavioral context.

4. Crossmodal plasticity

As sensory organs are highly specialized, the cooperative interplay of sensory systems improves perception through multimodal integration enhancing reliability of the information conveyed by each sensory channel, all the more so when individuals are engaged in a perceptually complex behavioral context. Hence, it has been assumed for decades that multimodal integration favors crossmodal plasticity and promotes functional compensation following partial or total deprivation of a sensory modality. Accordingly, a cortical area deprived of its dominant sensory input exhibits an increased responsiveness to stimulation of other modalities, thereby changing its functional tuning. There are a wealth of electrophysiological, neuroimaging and behavioral studies carried out in deaf and blind subjects that have provided convincing evidence for intersensory substitution in deprived cortical areas and experience-dependent reorganization in the areas taking over the defective sensory modality [59–63]. The plasticity mechanisms mediating these changes have also been extensively investigated, with a focus on the ingrowth of novel heteromodal projections or the unmasking of already existing heteromodal inputs. In this chapter, we focus the discussion on crossmodal plasticity occurring within primary areas.

4.1 Heteromodal recruitment of deprived visual cortex

4.1.1 Visual to somatosensory substitution

Capacity for tactile perception to substitute, at least partly, for the loss of vision has long been established [64]. Neuroimaging studies have provided evidence that the occipital visual cortex can be recruited by tactile tasks in blind subjects. For example, a PET study revealed that blind subjects display activation of primary and secondary visual cortical areas during tactile discrimination tasks, in contrast to sighted subjects who exhibited deactivation (i.e., decreased regional cerebral blood flow) in these areas [65]. In addition, this study showed that tactile recruitment of the visual cortex may be task-specific, since a non-discrimination tactile task did not activate V1 in either the blind or sighted subjects. This finding was corroborated in a fMRI study which also showed that electrical stimulation of the hand reading Braille dots did not evoke activation in the visual cortex, suggesting that the tactile recruitment in the visual cortex may result from high-order supramodal processing [66]. Interestingly, transcranial magnetic stimulation (TMS) of the occipital visual cortex overlying Brodmann areas 17, 18 and 19 in early-onset blind subjects, while they were identifying Braille or embossed Roman letters, was found to distort tactile perception [67]. By contrast, no such impairment of tactile performance was observed in sighted subjects. Furthermore, V1 was not only strongly activated during Braille reading, but also during Braille writing from memory in the most foveal part of V1 [68]. However, activation of occipital areas during Braille reading was not found in late-onset blind subjects, and their stimulation by TMS did not disrupt braille reading [69]. This report is at variance with other studies showing V1 activation in late onset blind subjects during braille reading [70, 71]. Individuals who lost sight as adults, and subsequently learned Braille, still exhibit activity in V1, although the spatial extent of the activation in the visual cortex is greater for those who became blind early in life [71]. Moreover, the early-onset blind subjects were found to display stronger activation in the occipital cortex contralateral to the hand used for reading Braille.

In late-blind patients with retinitis pigmentosa, vision deprivation leads to an elevated activation of the visual cortex in response to tactile stimuli during a discriminative task, with higher activation as the degree of vision loss was greater [72]. It is worth mentioning that even in normally sighted adults, five days of complete visual deprivation combined with intensive tactile training result in increased BOLD signal within the occipital cortex in response to tactile stimulation, hence reflecting visual areas engagement in the processing of non-visual information [73]. This crossmodal activation was reversed within 24 hours of removing the blindfold. Surprisingly, even after a short period of blindfolding (40-60 min), V1 activation was observed while the subjects performed a fine spatial tactile discrimination task [74]. Along the same lines, a one-week visual deprivation in juvenile mice was found to improve whisker function. This short period deprivation was sufficient to sharpen the tuning of layer 2/3 neurons in the barrel field of S1 [75].

Considering both the improvement in Braille character tactile discrimination after the five-day blindfolding period [73] and the impairment of Braille character recognition after disruption of the occipital cortex by TMS [67], it is reasonable to infer that crossmodal changes taking place in the visually deprived occipital cortex are behaviorally adaptive. A further argument stems from an interesting study showing that, when systematically stimulating the occipital cortex with single pulse TMS, early- and late -onset blind subjects have reported tactile sensations in the Braille-reading fingers, that were somatotopically mapped onto the visual cortex, whereas blindfolded sighted controls reported only phosphenes [76]. Further evidence for the adaptive function of tactile information processing in the visual cortex of early blind subjects comes from a study reporting the case of a proficient Braille reader blind from birth who was no longer able to read Braille (Braille alexia) after bilateral ischemic stroke to the occipital cortex, while somatosensory perception was otherwise unchanged [77]. The core evidence reported herein supports the view that the recruitment of V1 by somatosensory inputs in the context of compensatory behavioral strategy (Braille reading) accounts, at least in part, for the superior tactile perceptual abilities of blind people [67].

4.1.2 Visual to auditory substitution

Numerous studies have documented the fact that occipital cortical areas can be activated by auditory inputs in blind subjects (for reviews, see [60, 78]). For example, in the early-blind macaque, the occipital visual cortical areas were shown to respond to auditory stimulation [79]; Likewise, auditory responses in the visual cortex of neonatally enucleated rats have been recorded in a third of the V1 neurons recorded [80]. Contrary to a prevailing view, recent studies in late blind subjects have demonstrated that crossmodal plastic changes also occur in the adult. Sound change detection was found to recruit occipital cortical areas in individuals with both early- and late-onset blindness [81]. Further evidence was provided by a positron emission tomography (PET) study showing that visual cortical areas, including V1, were activated during auditory word processing in the congenitally blind and in subjects who had become blind after puberty [70].

There has been longstanding controversy about whether auditory signal processing can compensate for impaired accuracy of spatial representation in blind subjects. For example, fMRI studies have shown that, in early-blind people, V1 is activated during auditory detection and recognition [82] as well as during auditory localization tasks [83]. Early blind subjects are found to localize sound sources with a better accuracy than sighted subjects, in particular in monaural condition [84]. In this study, it was reported that subjects displaying a residual peripheral vision localized sound less precisely than sighted or totally blind subjects. Moreover, in blind individuals, experts at perceiving space through sound echoes using clicks (echolocators), evidence was found for a retinotopic-like mapping of sounds in V1 [85]. This finding indicates that the early visual area can be adapted to precisely remap spatial locations after visual loss. It is worth mentioning that the degree of retinotopic-like mapping of sound echoes was positively associated with echo localization ability [85]. Overall, the findings reported above strongly suggest that crossmodal substitution leading to a functional remapping of sensory and cognitive functions in the deprived cortex depends upon the extent of sensory loss and the nature of the task to be compensated for. It turns out that the crossmodal substitution is limited by the degree of functional overlap or cooperativity between sensory systems. It is worth mentioning a fMRI investigation using auditory discrimination in the congenitally blind with a focus on the effective connectivity between different cortical and thalamic regions via dynamic causal modeling [86]. The data showed a clear enhancement of BOLD responses in bilateral V1 during the auditory task, hence corroborating a previous study [87], and provided evidence for stronger corticocortical effective connectivity from A1 to V1 in blind than in sighted subjects. Furthermore, a combination of dynamic causal modeling with Bayesian selection has demonstrated that auditory-driven activity in the occipital cortex of the congenitally blind is best explained by direct feed-forward connections from A1 to V1, whereas it relies more on indirect feedback inputs from parietal regions in the late-onset blind subjects [88]. This study suggests that visual deprivation during an early critical period induces a crossmodal plasticity under the form of a transfer of spatial processing competency to a non-visual modality in the deprived cortex.

4.2 Heteromodal recruitment of deprived auditory cortex

In this section, we will not distinguish data related to the recruitment of the deprived auditory cortex by somatosensory or visual modalities. As found in blind subjects, animal and human studies have provided ample evidence of crossmodal plasticity after hearing loss. Recruitment of the deprived auditory cortical areas during somatosensory and visual stimulation in deaf individuals was repeatedly observed in higher-order auditory cortex (for review: [60, 89]). By contrast, it remains controversial whether the deafferented primary auditory cortex may be activated by spared sensory modalities. An electrophysiological investigation in congenitally deaf cats failed to detect crossmodal responses to visual or somatosensory stimuli in A1 [90]. Moreover, inactivation of A1 by cooling had no obvious effect on behaviorally-tested visual functions in the congenitally deaf cats [91]. Yet, after early destruction of cochlear receptors, photic stimulation was found to elicit neural activation in A1 of mature cats [92]. However, this crossmodal modification was observed after early-onset deprivation (one week), a period in which primary cortical areas are not yet well defined, but not after late-onset (2 month-old cats) auditory deprivation. Nevertheless, there is evidence in deaf cats for alteration in the pattern of heteromodal thalamocortical and corticocortical projections from somatosensory and visual areas to A1 [93]. Somatosensory projections were more prominent in early- and late-onset deaf animals, whereas projections originating from the visual areas were less apparent in the late-onset than early-onset deaf animals. These findings suggest that crossmodal anatomical plasticity in the deprived auditory cortex differs depending on the age of deafness onset and sensory modality. Furthermore, in early-deaf cats, increased projections from neighboring visual and somatosensory areas to the core auditory cortex including A1 and the surrounding anterior auditory field (AAF) have been described [94]. Interestingly, a study combining electrophysiological recording with cortical myelo-architecture description in congenitally deaf mice showed that the visual and somatosensory spatial domains had taken over auditory domains within A1 and AAF [95]. This finding demonstrates extensive re-specification of cortical fields following auditory loss. In addition, in early deafened ferrets, recordings from single-units in the core auditory cortex showed that 72% were activated by somatosensory stimulation, compared to 1% in hearing controls [96]. In adult-deafened ferrets, extensive crossmodal reorganization of core auditory cortex was also described, which was characterized by a consistent somatosensory conversion in neuron responsiveness within 16 days after deafening [97], thus demonstrating that crossmodal plasticity can also occur after the period of sensory system maturation. These data suggest that subthreshold tactile inputs found in hearing animals can transform into suprathreshold responses in adult deafened animals. In this regard, it is worth mentioning that somatosensory inputs to the core auditory cortex represent the majority of non-auditory effects in hearing ferrets [96]. This specificity may be due to the greater functional similarities between somatosensory and auditory modalities regarding temporal precision underlying frequency percept (e.g. vibrotactile stimulations), compared to that between audition and vision.

The recruitment of A1 for the processing of visual stimuli was also revealed by fMRI investigations in congenitally or early deaf subjects [98–100]. Moreover, in adult-onset single-sided deafness (SSD), seeded functional connectivity of visual cortices revealed enhancement in visual areas and reduction in auditory regions, suggesting adaptive functional modifications of the visual network [101]. Furthermore, V1 seeds demonstrated increased connectivity in multiple regions, including those dedicated to speech (inferior parietal lobule) or somatosensory processing (postcentral gyrus). It is also noticeable that activation of A1 was observed in deaf subjects with total hearing loss during sign language tasks, but not in subjects with residual hearing ability [102], suggesting that this crossmodal plasticity depends on the extent of hearing loss. Additional evidence of compensatory functional changes comes from the observation that congenitally deaf cats, compared with hearing cats, have superior localization abilities in the peripheral visual field and lower visual movement detection thresholds [91]. In this study, reversible deactivation of posterior auditory cortex was found to selectively eliminate superior visual localization abilities, whereas deactivation of the dorsal auditory cortex eliminated superior visual motion detection. It is of interest that measuring the fMRI signal changes in response to spatially co-registered visual, somatosensory and bimodal stimuli, the visual responses which were stronger in congenitally deaf than hearing adults, appeared to be weaker than those elicited by somatosensory stimulation [103]. This is consistent with the above-mentioned finding on the prevalence of somatosensory over visual inputs in the core auditory cortex [96]. Congenital deafness was also found to enhance the accuracy of suprathreshold tactile change detection, while tactile frequency discrimination thresholds tended to be reduced [104]. Beyond noticeable interspecies differences in the potential of crossmodal reorganization [61], the aforementioned studies highlight that deprived auditory sensory cortical areas become re-engaged in the processing of remaining sensory modalities.

5. Compensatory plasticity in the remaining sensory cortices

The crossmodal plasticity concept has been extended by studies demonstrating that the loss of one sense induces substantial alteration in remaining sensory cortical areas leading to experience-dependent refinement of neuronal responses. The so-called compensatory plasticity is conceived as underlying higher than normal perceptual abilities. However, it is notable that the available experimental evidence of compensatory plasticity is scarce compared to that documenting crossmodal plasticity. Nonetheless, changes involving processing of visual signals have been described following somatosensory and auditory deprivation. In adult mice, partial somatosensory deprivation (bilateral removal of macro-whiskers) lasting 12 days induced a massive increase of V1 responses elicited by weak visual stimuli, which was accompanied by a marked improvement of spatial frequency and contrast tuning (40%) of V1 neurons, as revealed by intrinsic signal imaging [105]. It is noteworthy that visual acuity and contrast sensitivity determined in behavioral tasks in individual animals improved by 40% and 60%, respectively, i.e., similarly to what was observed in V1. In addition, auditory deprivation in adult mice induces salient changes in visually evoked responses in V1, with improvement of spatial frequency and contrast tuning [106]. Conversely, visual deprivation (one week of dark exposure) in adult mice leads to improved frequency selectivity as well as increased frequency tuning and intensity discrimination performance of A1 neurons [107]. Collectively, these studies show that compensatory plasticity can develop after short-term deprivation in adult sensory cortices and highlight the fact that deprivation of one sense rapidly refines sensory processing in remaining cortical areas, while improving sensory guided behavior.

6. Putative mechanisms mediating crossmodal plasticity

A review of the literature indicates that a plethora of neuronal mechanisms such as stabilization of transient connections, unmasking of silent synapses, reinforcement/reweighing of subthreshold connections, structural changes such as axonal sprouting and dendritic arborization remodeling, are all putative mechanisms of crossmodal plasticity [59, 61, 108, 109]. Despite the wealth of data, these cellular and molecular mechanisms remain poorly understood. All these neural mechanisms may operate in subcortical, thalamocortical, as well as primary and associative cortical areas.

To offer some insight into the neural mechanisms underpinning crossmodal plasticity, we will mention a limited sample of studies. For example, concerning changes within the primary sensory areas, cross-modal synaptic plasticity is thought to involve LTP/LTD mechanisms [108]. Furthermore, the improved frequency selectivity and intensity discrimination of A1 neurons following visual deprivation in adult mice was attributed to a strengthening of thalamocortical synapses in A1, but not in V1 [107]. In addition, this deprivation was found to potentiate layer 4 to layer 2/3 synapses in A1 [110]. Such a selective effect suggests that the adult brain retains the capability for crossmodal changes, whereas this capability is absent or very limited within a sensory modality. This view seems to be corroborated by the observation that visual deprivation via lid suture that allows residual visual activity is sufficient to trigger a scaling-up of excitatory synapses in the S1 barrel fields. By contrast, this mild deprivation fails to trigger such a scaling up in V1 which requires a complete loss of visual activity [111]. Furthermore, dark rearing for 1 week in young rats (4-week-old) produces changes in synaptic function in S1 and A1. It was then hypothesized that the scaling-up of V1 synapses might allow recruitment of V1 for processing previously subthreshold inputs carrying tactile or auditory information, while scaling-down of S1 and A1 synapses may sharpen neuronal properties for enhanced perception thus constituting a basis for a sensory compensation [108, 111]. In these somatosensory and auditory cortical areas, decreased amplitudes of AMPA receptor-mediated excitatory transmission in layer 2/3 pyramidal neurons were observed, whereas opposite effects were recorded in the deprived visual cortex [112]. These changes were rapidly reversed after 2 days of light exposure. This study raises the question of whether the crossmodal plasticity induced in somatosensory cortex is due to the altered cortical processing of tactile inputs engaging cortico-cortical pathways or to differences in tactile experience involving thalamocortical projections. In addition to these alterations in the strength of intracortical synapses, visual deprivation (dark exposure for 6–8 days) was found to produce a refinement of intra- and inter-laminar functional circuitry in A1, in the adult mouse. Using *in vitro* whole-cell patch recordings in thalamocortical slices from auditory cortex, it was shown that this period of dark exposure can refine ascending and intralaminar excitatory and inhibitory circuits to layer 2/3 neurons [113], as well as interlaminar excitatory and inhibitory connections from layer 2/3 to layer 4 neurons [114]. Mathematical modeling of the data shows that the observed refinements increase the firing reliability of sound-evoked responses [113]. Visual deprivation in the rat was found to produce an increase in extracellular serotonin levels facilitating synaptic strengthening at layer 4 to layer 2/3 synapses in the barrel cortex [75]. Beyond this local effect, crossmodal plasticity may also engage large-scale modulatory mechanisms mediated, for instance, by the serotoninergic system to orchestrate cortical reorganization in relation with arousal and attention shift from the deprived to the intact sense [115, 116]. It is also worth mentioning that a positive correlation was depicted between behavioral performances in auditory and tactile tasks, and both the myelination of intracortical neurons and gray matter concentration measured in the occipital cortical areas of early-blind adults [117].

Even though crossmodal plasticity was demonstrated in early and late deprived subjects, the age of sensory loss onset seems to play a crucial role in the mechanisms involved [118]. In the case of congenitally or early sensory loss, primary cortical areas may retune their functional specificity based on the maintenance, during the developmental period, of intermodal projecting axons that would have otherwise been pruned. By contrast, in the case of late deprivation, crossmodal plasticity may rely on the remodeling and strengthening of pre-existing inputs in the deprived or spared cortical areas. Species-specificity also accounts for crossmodal plasticity, as primary-to primary areas connectivity changes have been show to occur in rodent, but less consistently in higher order species [61].

7. Conclusion

Collectively, the reported studies on crossmodal interplay and plasticity in primary cortical areas after sensory loss challenge the view that multisensory integration and plasticity only exists in high-order cortical areas. Future studies should investigate how the crossmodal substitution effects shown in the deprived primary areas contribute to the high-order cortices plasticity after a sensory loss and more generally promote adaptive behavioral performances through functional compensation. In this respect, it will be important to decipher the neural mechanisms underpinning the necessary rebalancing of bottom-up and top-down regulatory influences in order to improve neuro-rehabilitative procedures.

Abbreviations

A1, V1, S1	primary auditory, visual and somatosensory areas of the neocortex respectively
V2	secondary visual cortical area
1/3b	areas 1 and 3b of the primary somatosensory cortex

Author details

Christian Xerri* and Yoh'i Zennou-Azogui
Aix Marseille Université-CNRS, Laboratoire de Neurosciences Sensorielles et Cognitives (LNSC), UMR 7260, Marseille, France

*Address all correspondence to: christian.xerri@univ-amu.fr

References

[1] Falchier A, Clavagnier S, Barone P, et al. Anatomical Evidence of Multimodal Integration in Primate Striate Cortex. Journal of Neuroscience 2002; 22: 5749-5759. DOI:10.1523/JNEUROSCI.22-13-05749.2002

[2] Cappe C, Barone P. Heteromodal connections supporting multisensory integration at low levels of cortical processing in the monkey. European Journal of Neuroscience 2005; 22: 2886-2902. DOI:10.1016/j.heares.2009.04.017

[3] Bizley JK, Nodal FR, Bajo VM, et al. Physiological and Anatomical Evidence for Multisensory Interactions in Auditory Cortex. Cerebral Cortex 2007; 17: 2172-2189. DOI:10.1093/cercor/bhl128

[4] Ghazanfar A, Schroeder C. Is neocortex essentially multisensory? Trends in Cognitive Sciences 2006; 10: 278-285. DOI:10.1016/j.tics.2006.04.008

[5] Teichert M, Bolz J. How Senses Work Together: Cross-Modal Interactions between Primary Sensory Cortices. Neural Plasticity 2018; 2018: 1-11. DOI:10.1155/2018/5380921

[6] Henschke JU, Noesselt T, Scheich H, et al. Possible anatomical pathways for short-latency multisensory integration processes in primary sensory cortices. Brain Structure and Function 2015; 220: 955-977. DOI:10.1007/s00429-013-0694-4

[7] Hall AJ, Lomber SG. Auditory cortex projections target the peripheral field representation of primary visual cortex. Experimental Brain Research 2008; 190: 413-430. DOI:10.1007/s00221-008-1485-7

[8] Charbonneau V, Laramée M-E, Boucher V, et al. Cortical and subcortical projections to primary visual cortex in anophthalmic, enucleated and sighted mice: Connections of primary visual cortex in blind mice. European Journal of Neuroscience 2012; 36: 2949-2963. DOI:10.1111/j.1460-9568.2012.08215.x

[9] Massé IO, Ross S, Bronchti G, et al. Asymmetric Direct Reciprocal Connections Between Primary Visual and Somatosensory Cortices of the Mouse. Cerebral Cortex 2016; 1-18. DOI:10.1093/cercor/bhw239

[10] Iurilli G, Ghezzi D, Olcese U, et al. Sound-Driven Synaptic Inhibition in Primary Visual Cortex. Neuron 2012; 73: 814-828. DOI:10.1016/j.neuron.2011.12.026

[11] Sieben K, Roder B, Hanganu-Opatz IL. Oscillatory Entrainment of Primary Somatosensory Cortex Encodes Visual Control of Tactile Processing. Journal of Neuroscience 2013; 33: 5736-5749. DOI:10.1523/JNEUROSCI.4432-12.2013

[12] Schroeder CE, Lindsley RW, Specht C, et al. Somatosensory Input to Auditory Association Cortex in the Macaque Monkey. Journal of Neurophysiology 2001; 85: 1322-1327. DOI:10.1152/jn.2001.85.3.1322

[13] Brosch M. Nonauditory Events of a Behavioral Procedure Activate Auditory Cortex of Highly Trained Monkeys. Journal of Neuroscience 2005; 25: 6797-6806. DOI:10.1523/JNEUROSCI.1571-05.2005

[14] Kayser C, Petkov CI, Logothetis NK. Visual Modulation of Neurons in Auditory Cortex. Cerebral Cortex 2008; 18: 1560-1574. DOI:10.1093/cercor/bhm187

[15] Giard MH, Peronnet F. Auditory-Visual Integration during Multimodal Object Recognition in Humans: A Behavioral and Electrophysiological Study. Journal of Cognitive

Neuroscience 1999; 11: 473-490. DOI:10.1162/089892999563544

[16] Foxe JJ, Morocz IA, Murray MM, et al.Multisensoryauditory–somatosensory interactions in early cortical processing revealed by high-density electrical mapping. Cognitive Brain Research 2000; 7.

[17] Murray MM, Molholm S, Michel CM, et al. Grabbing Your Ear: Rapid Auditory–Somatosensory Multisensory Interactions in Low-level Sensory Cortices Are Not Constrained by Stimulus Alignment. Cerebral Cortex 2005; 15: 963-974. DOI:10.1093/cercor/bhh197

[18] Felleman DJ, Van Essen DC. Distributed Hierarchical Processing in the Primate Cerebral Cortex. Cerebral Cortex 1991; 1: 1-47. DOI:10.1093/cercor/1.1.1

[19] Salin PA, Bullier J. Corticocortical connections in the visual system: structure and function. Physiological Reviews 1995; 75: 107-154. DOI:10.1152/physrev.1995.75.1.107

[20] Schroeder CE, Foxe JJ. The timing and laminar profile of converging inputs to multisensory areas of the macaque neocortex. Cognitive Brain Research 2002; 14: 187-198. DOI:10.1016/S0926-6410(02)00073-3

[21] Foxe JJ, Schroeder CE. The case for feedforward multisensory convergence during early cortical processing: NeuroReport 2005; 16: 419-423. DOI:10.1097/00001756-200504040-00001

[22] Ibrahim LA, Mesik L, Ji X, et al. Cross-Modality Sharpening of Visual Cortical Processing through Layer-1-Mediated Inhibition and Disinhibition. Neuron 2016; 89: 1031-1045. DOI:10.1016/j.neuron.2016.01.027

[23] Meijer GT, Montijn JS, Pennartz CMA, et al. Audiovisual Modulation in Mouse Primary Visual Cortex Depends on Cross-Modal Stimulus Configuration and Congruency. Journal of Neuroscience 2017; 37: 8783-8796. DOI:10.1523/JNEUROSCI.0468-17.2017

[24] Wang Y, Celebrini S, Trotter Y, et al. Visuo-auditory interactions in the primary visual cortex of the behaving monkey: Electrophysiological evidence. BMC Neuroscience 2008; 9: 79. DOI:10.1186/1471-2202-9-79

[25] Kayser C, Logothetis NK, Panzeri S. Visual Enhancement of the Information Representation in Auditory Cortex. Current Biology 2010; 20: 19-24. DOI:10.1016/j.cub.2009.10.068

[26] Morrill RJ, Hasenstaub AR. Visual Information Present in Infragranular Layers of Mouse Auditory Cortex. Journal of Neuroscience 2018; 38: 2854-2862. DOI:10.1523/JNEUROSCI.3102-17.2018

[27] Engel AK, Senkowski D, Schneider TR. Multisensory Integration through Neural Coherence. In: Murray MM, Wallace MT, editors. The Neural Bases of Multisensory Processes. Boca Raton (FL): CRC Press/Taylor & Francis; 2012. Chapter 7. PMID: 22593880.

[28] Lakatos P, Chen C-M, O'Connell MN, et al. Neuronal Oscillations and Multisensory Interaction in Primary Auditory Cortex. Neuron 2007; 53: 279-292. DOI:10.1016/j.neuron.2006.12.011

[29] Fu K-MG, Johnston TA, Shah AS, et al. Auditory Cortical Neurons Respond to Somatosensory Stimulation. Journal of Neuroscience 2003; 23: 7510-7515. DOI:10.1523/JNEUROSCI.23-20-07510.2003

[30] Rauschecker JP. Parallel Processing in the Auditory Cortex of Primates. Audiology and Neurotology 1998; 3: 86-103. DOI:10.1159/000013784

[31] Kaas JH, Hackett TA, Tramo MJ. Auditory processing in primate cerebral cortex. Current Opinion in Neurobiology 1999, 9:164-170

[32] Kayser C, Petkov CI, Augath M, et al. Integration of Touch and Sound in Auditory Cortex. Neuron 2005; 48: 373-384. DOI:10.1016/j.neuron.2005.09.018

[33] Eck J, Kaas AL, Goebel R. Crossmodal interactions of haptic and visual texture information in early sensory cortex. NeuroImage 2013; 75: 123-135. DOI:10.1016/j.neuroimage.2013.02.075

[34] Sathian K, Lacey S, Stilla R, et al. Dual pathways for haptic and visual perception of spatial and texture information. NeuroImage 2011; 57: 462-475. DOI:10.1016/j.neuroimage.2011.05.001

[35] Kuehn E, Mueller K, Turner R, et al. The functional architecture of S1 during touch observation described with 7 T fMRI. Brain Structure and Function 2014; 219: 119-140. DOI:10.1007/s00429-012-0489-z

[36] Dykes RW. Parallel Processing of Somatosensory Information: A Theory. Brain Research Review 1983; 6: 47-115.

[37] Jones EG. GABAergic Neurons and Their Role in Cortical Plasticity in Primates. Cerebral Cortex 1993; 3: 361-372. DOI:10.1093/cercor/3.5.361-a

[38] Cardini F, Longo MR, Haggard P. Vision of the Body Modulates Somatosensory Intracortical Inhibition. Cerebral Cortex 2011; 21: 2014-2022. DOI:10.1093/cercor/bhq267

[39] Kuehn E, Haggard P, Villringer A, et al. Visually-Driven Maps in Area 3b. Journal of Neuroscience 2018; 38: 1295-1310. DOI:10.1523/JNEUROSCI.0491-17.2017

[40] Brandt T, Dieterich M. Thalamocortical network: a core structure for integrative multimodal vestibular functions. Current Opinion in Neurology 2019; 32: 154-164. DOI:10.1097/WCO.0000000000000638

[41] Lopez C. The vestibular system: balancing more than just the body. Current Opinion in Neurology 2016; 29: 74-83.

[42] Lopez C, Blanke O. The thalamocortical vestibular system in animals and humans. Brain Research Reviews 2011; 67: 119-146. DOI:10.1097/WCO.0000000000000286

[43] Rancz EA, Moya J, Drawitsch F, et al. Widespread Vestibular Activation of the Rodent Cortex. Journal of Neuroscience 2015; 35: 5926-5934. DOI:10.1523/JNEUROSCI.1869-14.2015

[44] Leong ATL, Gu Y, Chan Y-S, et al. Optogenetic fMRI interrogation of brain-wide central vestibular pathways. Proceedings of the National Academy of Sciences USA 2019; 116: 10122-10129. DOI:10.1073/pnas.1812453116

[45] Facchini J, Rastoldo G, Péricat D, et al. Unilateral vestibular neurectomy induces a remodeling of somatosensory cortical maps. Progress in Neurobiology (in press).

[46] Magnin M, Kennedy H. Anatomical evidence of a third ascending vestibular pathway involving the ventral lateral geniculate nucleus and the intralaminar nuclei of the cat. Brain Research 1979; 171: 523-529. DOI:10.1016/0006-8993(79)91056-4

[47] Kotchabhakdi N, Rinvik E, Walberg F, et al. The vestibulothalamic projections in the cat studied by retrograde axonal transport of horseradish peroxidase. Experimental Brain Research; 40. Epub ahead of print November 1980. DOI:10.1007/BF00236149

[48] Alloway KD, Rosenthal P, Burton H. Quantitative measurements of receptive field changes during antagonism of GABAergic transmission in primary somatosensory cortex of cats. Experimental Brain Research; 78. Epub ahead of print December 1989. DOI:10.1007/BF00230239

[49] Dykes RW, Landry P, Metherate R, et al. Functional role of GABA in cat primary somatosensory cortex: shaping receptive fields of cortical neurons. Journal of Neurophysiology 1984; 52: 1066-1093. DOI:10.1152/jn.1984.52.6.1066

[50] Tremere L, Hicks TP, Rasmusson DD. Role of Inhibition in Cortical Reorganization of the Adult Raccoon Revealed by Microiontophoretic Blockade of GABA $_A$ Receptors. Journal of Neurophysiology 2001; 86: 94-103. DOI:10.1152/jn.2001.86.1.94

[51] Kyriazi HT, Carvell GE, Brumberg JC, et al. Quantitative effects of GABA and bicuculline methiodide on receptive field properties of neurons in real and simulated whisker barrels. Journal of Neurophysiology 1996; 75: 547-560. DOI:10.1152/jn.1996.75.2.547

[52] Teichert M, Bolz J. Simultaneous intrinsic signal imaging of auditory and visual cortex reveals profound effects of acute hearing loss on visual processing. NeuroImage 2017; 159: 459-472. DOI:10.1016/j.neuroimage.2017.07.037

[53] Lippert MT, Takagaki K, Kayser C, et al. Asymmetric Multisensory Interactions of Visual and Somatosensory Responses in a Region of the Rat Parietal Cortex. PLoS ONE 2013; 8: e63631. DOI:10.1371/journal.pone.0063631

[54] Olcese U, Iurilli G, Medini P. Cellular and Synaptic Architecture of Multisensory Integration in the Mouse Neocortex. Neuron 2013; 79: 579-593. DOI:10.1016/j.neuron.2013.06.010

[55] Takagaki K, Zhang C, Wu J-Y, et al. Crossmodal propagation of sensory-evoked and spontaneous activity in the rat neocortex. Neuroscience Letters 2008; 431: 191-196. DOI:10.1016/j.neulet.2007.11.069

[56] Caron-Guyon J, Corbo J, Zennou-Azogui Y, et al. Neuronal Encoding of Multisensory Motion Features in the Rat Associative Parietal Cortex. Cerebral Cortex 2020; 30: 5372-5386. DOI:10.1093/cercor/bhaa118

[57] Sereno MI, Huang R-S. Multisensory maps in parietal cortex. Current Opinion in Neurobiology 2014; 24: 39-46. DOI:10.1016/j.conb.2013.08.014

[58] Huang R-S, Sereno MI. Multisensory and sensorimotor maps. In: Handbook of Clinical Neurology. Elsevier, pp. 141-161. DOI:10.1016/B978-0-444-63622-5.00007-3

[59] Bavelier D, Neville HJ. Cross-modal plasticity: where and how? Nature Review Neuroscience 2002; 3: 443-452. DOI: 10.1038/nrn848.

[60] Heimler B, Weisz N, Collignon O. Revisiting the adaptive and maladaptive effects of crossmodal plasticity. Neuroscience 2014; 283: 44-63. DOI: 10.1016/j.neuroscience.2014.08.003.

[61] Meredith MA, Lomber SG. Species-dependent role of crossmodal connectivity among the primary sensory cortices. Hearing Research 2017; 343: 83-91. DOI: 10.1016/j.heares.2016.05.014.

[62] Singh AK, Phillips F, Merabet LB, et al. Why Does the Cortex Reorganize after Sensory Loss? Trends in Cognitive Sciences 2018; 22: 569-582. DOI: 10.1016/j.tics.2018.04.004.

[63] Bell L, Wagels L, Neuschaefer-Rube C, et al. The Cross-Modal Effects of Sensory Deprivation on Spatial and Temporal Processes in Vision and Audition: A Systematic Review on Behavioral and Neuroimaging Research since 2000. Neural Plasticity 2019; 2019: 1-21. DOI: 10.1155/2019/9603469.

[64] Bach-y-Rita P. *Brain Mechanisms in Sensory Substitution*, Academic Press New York:1972.

[65] Sadato N, Pascual-Leone A, Grafman J, et al. Activation of the primary visual cortex by Braille reading in blind subjects. Nature 1996; 380: 526-528. DOI: 10.1038/380526a0.

[66] Gizewski ER, Gasser T, de Greiff A, et al. Cross-modal plasticity for sensory and motor activation patterns in blind subjects. NeuroImage 2003; 19: 968-975. DOI: 10.1016/s1053-8119(03)00114-9.

[67] Cohen LG, Celnik P, Pascual-Leone A, et al. Functional relevance of cross-modal plasticity in blind humans. Nature 1997; 389: 180-183. DOI: 10.1038/38278.

[68] Likova LT, Tyler CW, Cacciamani L, et al. The Cortical Network for Braille Writing in the Blind. Electronic Imaging 2016; 2016: 1-6. DOI: 10.2352/ISSN.2470-1173.2016.16.HVEI-095.

[69] Cohen LG, Weeks RA, Sadato N, et al. Period of susceptibility for cross-modal plasticity in the blind. Annals of Neurology. 1999; 45(4):451-460. DOI: 10.1002/1531-8249(199904)45:4<451::aid-ana6>3.0.co;2-b.

[70] Buchel C. Different activation patterns in the visual cortex of late and congenitally blind subjects. Brain 1998; 121: 409-419. DOI: 10.1093/brain/121.3.409.

[71] Burton H, Snyder AZ, Diamond JB, et al. Adaptive Changes in Early and Late Blind: A fMRI Study of Verb Generation to Heard Nouns. Journal of Neurophysiology 2002; 88: 3359-3371. DOI: 10.1152/jn.00129.2002.

[72] Cunningham SI, Weiland JD, Pinglei Bao, et al. Visual cortex activation induced by tactile stimulation in late-blind individuals with retinitis pigmentosa. In: 2011 Annual International Conference of the IEEE Engineering in Medicine and Biology Society. Boston, MA: IEEE, pp. 2841-2844. DOI: 10.1109/IEMBS.2011.6090785.

[73] Merabet LB, Hamilton R, Schlaug G, et al. Rapid and Reversible Recruitment of Early Visual Cortex for Touch. PLoS ONE 2008; 3: e3046. DOI: 10.1371/journal.pone.0003046.

[74] Merabet LB, Swisher JD, McMains SA, et al. Combined Activation and Deactivation of Visual Cortex During Tactile Sensory Processing. Journal of Neurophysiology 2007; 97: 9. DOI: 10.1152/jn.00806.2006.

[75] Jitsuki S, Takemoto K, Kawasaki T, et al. Serotonin Mediates Cross-Modal Reorganization of Cortical Circuits. Neuron 2011; 69: 780-792. DOI: 10.1016/j.neuron.2011.01.016.

[76] Ptito M, Fumal A, de Noordhout AM, et al. TMS of the occipital cortex induces tactile sensations in the fingers of blind Braille readers. Experimental Brain Research 2008; 184: 193-200. DOI: 10.1007/s00221-007-1091-0.

[77] Hamilton R, Keenan JP, Catala M, et al. Alexia for Braille following bilateral occipital stroke in an early blind woman: NeuroReport 2000; 11: 237-240. DOI: 10.1097/00001756-200002070-00003.

[78] Merabet LB, Pascual-Leone A. Neural reorganization following sensory loss: the opportunity of change. Nature

Review Neuroscience 2010; 11: 44-52. DOI: 10.1038/nrn2758.

[79] Wang R, Wu L, Tang Z, et al. Visual cortex and auditory cortex activation in early binocularly blind macaques: A BOLD-fMRI study using auditory stimuli. Biochemical and Biophysical Research Communications 2017; 485: 796-801. DOI: 10.1016/j.bbrc.2017.02.133.

[80] Piché M, Chabot N, Bronchti G, et al. Auditory responses in the visual cortex of neonatally enucleated rats. Neuroscience 2007; 145: 1144-1156. DOI: 10.1016/j.neuroscience.2006.12.050.

[81] Kujala T, Huotilainen M, Sinkkonen J, et al. Visual cortex activation in blind humans during sound discrimination. Neuroscience Letters 1995; 183: 143-146. DOI: 10.1016/0304-3940(94)11135-6.

[82] Arno P, De Volder AG, Vanlierde A, et al. Occipital Activation by Pattern Recognition in the Early Blind Using Auditory Substitution for Vision. NeuroImage 2001; 13: 632-645. DOI: 10.1006/nimg.2000.0731.

[83] Weeks R, Horwitz B, Aziz-Sultan A, et al. A Positron Emission Tomographic Study of Auditory Localization in the Congenitally Blind. Journal of Neuroscience 2000; 20: 2664-2672. DOI: 10.1523/JNEUROSCI.20-07-02664.2000.

[84] Lessard N, Paré M, Lepore F, et al. Early-blind human subjects localize sound sources better than sighted subjects. Nature 1998; 395: 278-280. DOI: 10.1038/26228.

[85] Norman LJ, Thaler L. Retinotopic-like maps of spatial sound in primary 'visual' cortex of blind human echolocators. Proceedings of the Royal Society of Biology 2019; 286: 20191910. DOI: 10.1098/rspb.2019.1910.

[86] Klinge C, Eippert F, Roder B, et al. Corticocortical Connections Mediate Primary Visual Cortex Responses to Auditory Stimulation in the Blind. Journal of Neuroscience 2010; 30: 12798-12805. DOI: 10.1523/JNEUROSCI.2384-10.2010.

[87] Gougoux F, Belin P, Voss P, et al. Voice perception in blind persons: A functional magnetic resonance imaging study. Neuropsychologia 2009; 47: 2967-2974. DOI: 10.1016/j.neuropsychologia.2009.06.027.

[88] Collignon O, Dormal G, Albouy G, et al. Impact of blindness onset on the functional organization and the connectivity of the occipital cortex. Brain 2013; 136: 2769-2783. DOI: 10.1093/brain/awt176.

[89] Glick H, Sharma A. Cross-modal plasticity in developmental and age-related hearing loss: Clinical implications. Hearing Research 2017; 343: 191-201. DOI: 10.1016/j.heares.2016.08.012.

[90] Kral A, Schröder J-H, Klinke R, et al. Absence of cross-modal reorganization in the primary auditory cortex of congenitally deaf cats. Experimental Brain Research 2003; 153: 605-613. DOI: 10.1007/s00221-003-1609-z.

[91] Lomber SG, Meredith MA, Kral A. Cross-modal plasticity in specific auditory cortices underlies visual compensations in the deaf. Nature Neuroscience 2010; 13: 1421-1427. DOI: 10.1038/nn.2653.

[92] Rebillard G, Carlier E, Rebillard M, et al. Enhancement of visual responses on the primary auditory cortex of the cat after an early destruction of cochlear receptors. Brain

Research 1977; 129: 162-164. DOI: 10.1016/0006-8993(77)90980-5.

[93] Chabot N, Butler BE, Lomber SG. Differential modification of cortical and thalamic projections to cat primary auditory cortex following early- and late-onset deafness: Modified projections to A1 following deafness. Journal of Comparative Neurology 2015; 523: 2297-2320. DOI: 10.1002/cne.23790.

[94] Wong C, Chabot N, Kok MA, et al. Amplified somatosensory and visual cortical projections to a core auditory area, the anterior auditory field, following early- and late-onset deafness: Modified projections to AAF following deafness. Journal of Comparative Neurology 2015; 523: 1925-1947. DOI: 10.1002/cne.23771.

[95] Hunt DL, Yamoah EN, Krubitzer L. Multisensory plasticity in congenitally deaf mice: How are cortical areas functionally specified? Neuroscience 2006; 139: 1507-1524. DOI: 10.1016/j.neuroscience.2006.01.023.

[96] Meredith MA, Allman BL. Single-unit analysis of somatosensory processing in the core auditory cortex of hearing ferrets. Eur Journal of Neuroscience 2015; 41: 686-698. DOI: 10.1111/ejn.12828

[97] Allman BL, Keniston LP, Meredith MA. Adult deafness induces somatosensory conversion of ferret auditory cortex. Proceedings of the National Academy of Sciences USA 2009; 106(14):5925-5930. DOI: 10.1073/pnas.0809483106.

[98] Finney EM, Fine I, Dobkins KR. Visual stimuli activate auditory cortex in the deaf. Nature Neuroscience 2001; 4: 1171-1173. DOI: 10.1038/nn763.

[99] Fine I, Finney EM, Boynton GM, et al. Comparing the Effects of Auditory Deprivation and Sign Language within the Auditory and Visual Cortex. Journal of Cognitive Neuroscience 2005; 17: 1621-1637. DOI: 10.1162/089892905774597173.

[100] Scott GD, Karns CM, Dow MW, et al. Enhanced peripheral visual processing in congenitally deaf humans is supported by multiple brain regions, including primary auditory cortex. Frontiers in Human Neuroscience; 8. Epub ahead of print 26 March 2014. DOI: 10.3389/fnhum.2014.00177. DOI: 10.3389/fnhum.2014.00177.

[101] Shang Y, Hinkley LB, Cai C, et al. Cross-modal plasticity in adult single-sided deafness revealed by alpha band resting-state functional connectivity. NeuroImage 2020; 207: 116376. DOI: 10.1016/j.neuroimage.2019.116376.

[102] Lambertz N, Gizewski ER, de Greiff A, et al. Cross-modal plasticity in deaf subjects dependent on the extent of hearing loss. Cognitive Brain Research 2005; 25: 884-890. DOI: 10.1016/j.cogbrainres.2005.09.010.

[103] Karns CM, Dow MW, Neville HJ. Altered Cross-Modal Processing in the Primary Auditory Cortex of Congenitally Deaf Adults: A Visual-Somatosensory fMRI Study with a Double-Flash Illusion. Journal of Neuroscience 2012; 32(28):9626-9638. DOI: 10.1523/JNEUROSCI.6488-11.2012.

[104] Levänen S, Hamdorf D. Feeling vibrations: enhanced tactile sensitivity in congenitally deaf humans. Neuroscience Letters 2001; 301: 75-77. DOI: 10.1016/s0304-3940(01)01597-x.

[105] Teichert M, Isstas M, Wenig S, et al. Cross-modal refinement of visual performance after brief somatosensory deprivation in adult mice. European Journal of Neuroscience 2018; 47(2):184-191 DOI: 10.1111/ejn.13798.

[106] Teichert M, Liebmann L, Hübner CA, et al. Homeostatic plasticity and synaptic scaling in the adult mouse auditory cortex. Science Report 2017; 7: 17423. DOI: 10.1038/s41598-017-17711-5.

[107] Petrus E, Isaiah A, Jones AP, et al. Crossmodal Induction of Thalamocortical Potentiation Leads to Enhanced Information Processing in the Auditory Cortex. Neuron 2014; 81: 664-673. DOI: 10.1016/j.neuron.2013.11.023.

[108] Lee H-K, Whitt JL. Cross-modal synaptic plasticity in adult primary sensory cortices. Current Opinion in Neurobiology 2015; 35: 119-126. DOI: 10.1016/j.conb.2015.08.002.

[109] Macharadze T, Budinger E, Brosch M, et al. Early Sensory Loss Alters the Dendritic Branching and Spine Density of Supragranular Pyramidal Neurons in Rodent Primary Sensory Cortices. Frontiers in Neural Circuits 2019; 13: 61. DOI: 10.3389/fncir.2019.00061.

[110] Petrus E, Rodriguez G, Patterson R, et al. Vision Loss Shifts the Balance of Feedforward and Intracortical Circuits in Opposite Directions in Mouse Primary Auditory and Visual Cortices. Journal of Neuroscience 2015; 35: 8790-8801. DOI: 10.1523/JNEUROSCI.4975-14.2015.

[111] He K, Petrus E, Gammon N, et al. Distinct Sensory Requirements for Unimodal and Cross-Modal Homeostatic Synaptic Plasticity. Journal of Neuroscience 2012; 32: 8469-8474. DOI: 10.1523/JNEUROSCI.1424-12.2012.

[112] Goel A, Jiang B, Xu LW, et al. Cross-modal regulation of synaptic AMPA receptors in primary sensory cortices by visual experience. Nature Neuroscience 2006; 9: 1001-1003. DOI: 10.1038/nn1725.

[113] Meng X, Kao JPY, Lee H-K, et al. Visual Deprivation Causes Refinement of Intracortical Circuits in the Auditory Cortex. Cell Reports 2015; 12: 955-964. DOI: 10.1016/j.celrep.2015.07.018.

[114] Meng X, Kao JPY, Lee H-K, et al. Intracortical Circuits in Thalamorecipient Layers of Auditory Cortex Refine after Visual Deprivation. eNeuro 2017; 4: ENEURO.0092-17.2017. DOI: 10.1523/ENEURO.0092-17.2017.

[115] Macaluso E, Driver J. Spatial attention and crossmodal interactions between vision and touch. Neuropsychologia 2001; 39: 1304-1316. DOI: 10.1016/s0028-3932(01)00119-1.

[116] Dye MWG, Baril DE, Bavelier D. Which aspects of visual attention are changed by deafness? The case of the Attentional Network Test. Neuropsychologia 2007; 45: 1801-1811. DOI: 10.1016/j.neuropsychologia.2006.12.019.

[117] Voss P, Pike BG, Zatorre RJ. Evidence for both compensatory plastic and disuse atrophy-related neuroanatomical changes in the blind. Brain 2014; 137: 1224-1240. DOI: 10.1093/brain/awu030.

[118] Collignon O, Voss P, Lassonde M, et al. Cross-modal plasticity for the spatial processing of sounds in visually deprived subjects. Experimental Brain Research 2009; 192: 343-358. DOI: 10.1007/s00221-008-1553-z.